It's My Life and I'll do What I want

harvey r. manes

Authors Choice Press

New York Bloomington

It's My Life and I'll Do What I Want

Authors Choice Press
an imprint of iUniverse

iUniverse books may be ordered through booksellers or by contacting:

iUniverse
1663 Liberty Drive
Bloomington, IN 47403
www.iuniverse.com
1-800-Authors (1-800-288-4677)

Because of the dynamic nature of the Internet, any Web addresses or links
contained in this book may have changed since publication and may no longer be
valid. The views expressed in this work are solely those of the author and do not
necessarily reflect the views of the publisher, and the publisher hereby disclaims
any responsibility for them.

ISBN: 978-1-4502-0578-8 (pbk)

Printed in the United States of America

iUniverse rev. date: 1/18/10

PREFACE

Captivating, perceptive, narrative, brimming with levity, "It's My Life" is available to readers on Amazon and Barnes&Nobles, preserved in the original format and now in its 2nd printing due to extraordinary demand.

Be the first to read his recent follow-up entitled "Mamas Don't Let Your Babies Grow Up to be Doctors" which is an insightful exposition of our national healthcare crises with a particular focus on the medical profession.

C.C., writer

TABLE OF CONTENTS

ACKNOWLEDGEMENTS

On this page which I almost left out, I would like to express my appreciation to everyone who participated in my life. Without their presence there would be no book to write. Any resemblance to a real person was done intentionally. This book was written in a spirit of love and respect for all. No offense was intended.

I would like to thank my editors, mostly from the Manes clan, who would not let me rest until each word and punctuation was exactly right. I take no responsibility for any editorial mishaps. HM

CHAPTER 1: YOU MUST HAVE BEEN A BEAUTIFUL BABY

There comes a time in your life when you should get off the treadmill and examine who you are, where you came from and where you are going. "An unexamined life is not worth living" Socrates said over two thousand years ago. I am writing this memoir, not for money or fame (although I would not object to either), and not to talk about myself while on an ego trip, but rather to inform, enlighten, and entertain the reader, my family and friends. I hope the reader will be able to see himself in some of the events that I describe and come away with some insight or a laugh about his own life. I am writing for my family and friends so they will have a more complete picture of who I am, which in turn may inspire them to examine their own lives. I am also writing for myself so that when I am an old man and read this book, perhaps I will have a good laugh. Some may think I have chutzpah to believe anybody would be interested in this book. They may be right and should stop reading now! All others may continue.

After fifty years or half a century, I feel it is an appropriate time to record the events that have taken place thus far before they are forever forgotten. The fact that I am writing this at the start of a new millennium is no coincidence since according to the Kabbala, there are no coincidences--everything occurs for a reason. If I could only understand some of these reasons I would have saved a lot of time and money wasted on psychotherapy. Frequently the reason is hidden and only known on a cosmic level at a different time. Hopefully this is the halfway point of my life and is therefore the perfect time for writing this autobiography.

I hope to live at least another fifty years at which time I will write a sequel. I am determined to live the next half century with the same zest and fervor as the first. I did not go this far to wimp out for the rest of the journey. Not me! I want to experience as much as possible and drink in all the flavors of life for the short time that I am here. I also hope to continue to grow intellectually and learn more about myself. I believe we should strive to reach our full potential as human beings. This cannot be done, by sitting around and contemplating our navels. Since the Bible states that we are created in the image of God, we must also be omniscient and have an infinite capacity to grow (and if you believe that, I have a lakeside condo for sale in the Ozarks). If you are not at least trying to live up to your potential then you are wasting your life away.

This is a "rags to riches to reality" story which may now be a cliché, but it is surely unique. Perhaps a good place to start an autobiography is at the beginning, when I was born. Actually, I will break with tradition and start before I was born, while inside the belly of my pregnant mother. I would have started with conception but I do not have any information about that fateful night. I wish I knew what was on their minds when they united, but I have a feeling it was not me, I was an unplanned pleasure baby (sounds better than a mistake). As luck would have it, my father quickly became frightened by the rapid growth of his wife's stomach so decided to take a long vacation in sunny Florida. He left my mother to fend for herself during one of the worst winters in New York history, the blizzard of '47. The City had to dig itself out of two feet of snow, and my mother was forced to go on "home relief" (welfare). I often wish that he had taken me with him to Florida. I never learned what the fight was about that resulted in their separation, but this was a precursor of a very bumpy marriage.

My mother and father had met on the beach at Coney Island some five years before while my mother was pregnant and married to another man who was in the army and stationed in Texas. My mother was way ahead of her time when it came to getting divorced, but she was simply following in her mother's footsteps. Grandma Brown, who came to America when she was 18 years old, was divorced in 1925. I believe her picture is in the Guinness Book for one of the first divorces on record. I am not sure how many years she was married or why her marriage failed but she became a single mom of two young daughters, my mother Rose and my Aunt Sally. Although it is not genetic, I think divorce does run in families, and runs the marathon in my family.

I was born on a beautiful night on the charity ward at Maimonides Hospital, in Brooklyn, May 25, 1948. (I could have lied about the year but my children would take me to task). My mother frequently reminds me about how difficult the delivery was because they had to do an episiotomy (cut through vaginal tissue), and use forceps to get me out. I guess I found it pretty comfortable inside. Needless to say, in those days they routinely did an episiotomy and used forceps on all deliveries. I guess my mom wanted me to be in debt to her for giving birth to me. Forget about the mahzol that a child brings to a parent. I am still trying to get over the guilt complex she laid on me. This is one of the reasons I became a doctor. I needed to understand what the birthing process really involved so I could decide for myself how much in debt I should truly be to her. P.S. Mom, I did not ask to be born and if you did not want to go through such torture then you should have used birth control or abstinence. Recently I read a quote by Schopenhauer, a very pessimistic philosopher who states "it is probably better to have never been born". There are days when I feel he is right. However, these are vastly outnumbered by days when it feels great to be alive. Maybe he never experienced sunsets, walking on the beach, falling in love, and having kids. Oops! With regard to kids maybe he was right. To bad he couldn't take Prozac.

Six months after my birth I ended up in an orphanage. No, my parents did not die, but nobody I have asked seems to know why I was there. I cannot get a straight answer out of my mother, father, or anyone else. I am told that I should not be bothered by this event since it happened so many years ago, and I should get on with my life. If it happened to you, wouldn't you want to know why? It is a riddle wrapped in a mystery inside an enigma (one of my favorite quotes from Winston Churchill about the Soviet Union). Apparently, my mother was hospitalized in the psychiatric ward at Kings County Hospital for a period of time. I believe the embarrassment is what keeps the information under wraps. Another unresolved question is why didn't anybody else in the family take me in? I had a father, aunts, uncles, grandparents, etc. I can only assume they were too busy with their own lives. I have been told that I was a very well behaved baby. How would anyone know this if I were in an orphanage? I was also told that my mother could not handle the burden of taking care of me because she could not take care of herself. Pardon me if I was a burden.

I was told that the orphanage was not the Dickensian kind that you see in the movies with sadistic automatons beating up on little kids, but instead there were caring nurses doing the best they could. I like to believe that. I do have one memory about the orphanage but I sometimes wonder whether it is a true event or a dream. I was sitting at a table with an empty seat next to me when a beautiful girl approached. I got off my chair and removed the empty chair from under the table so that she could sit down. I have no idea where I learned this act of chivalry. I should ask a behavioral scientist whether or not this is learned or instinctive. Either way, what a gentleman I must have been at age two.

For whatever reason (maybe I was too old); I was removed from the or-phanage at age three and placed in a foster home. There was this adorable little blonde girl about 7 years old living there. This was my first encounter with an older woman. But despite all my charm and good looks I did not get to first base with her. Maybe, I didn't have enough money. However, she did teach me a valuable lesson on how to brush my teeth. I did not know that you were supposed to squeeze the toothpaste onto the brush. I thought you were supposed to eat the paste right out of the tube.

I stayed in the home for about a year and in what was the most amazing coincidence of my life, our paths crossed again twenty years later. While I was a resident at Kings County Hospital, I was assigned to the pulmonary ward. On the first day I knew I would like working there because as soon as I walked into the nursing station I spotted this beautiful blonde nurse. In general, the nurses at the hospital were nothing much to look at. This one stood out from the crowd and at first glance she looked at me slightly longer than the customary two seconds. Several days later she handed me a picture of a little boy and girl sitting on a stoop. I looked very closely at the little boy and after a short time I realized that it was me. And the pretty little girl was now a pretty grown-up nurse. She remembered my name and vaguely what I looked like and realized who I was. The picture brought back memo-ries that were buried in the deepest recesses of my mind. I had completely forgotten about that period of time, living in her house with her mother who I used to call Mommy Faye. Although I immediately gave her the extra re-spect due to an older sister, a part of me felt this was another opportunity to try to score. For good reason, she shot me down.

At age four I left the foster home and began a new life with my mother and father in a tiny walk up apartment in Bensonhurst, Brooklyn (a place where all the finest and most talented people in the world have their roots). Suddenly, without any warning, I became part of the Manes family. One day, my mother was sitting in the kitchen and called out my name "Harvey, come here". As I walked over to her I remembered asking myself "who is this strange woman and why am I in her house? Then I realized that this stranger was my mother and that I was supposed to love her. What an epiphany! At the time, I did not feel that fuzzy, warm feeling that I was supposed to feel. This was the first time that I felt guilt. Only many years later did I understand why I felt detached from her. I hardly knew who she was! Later, in medical school, while studying Freud, I found out how important the first three years are for normal psychological development. By not having the closeness of a mother during this period, severe damage can be done to the psyche. The textbooks state that a person with my background might grow up dysfunctional (possibly a criminal). No wonder why I turned out to be a psycho. However, I think in my case, it may have been better not being around my neurotic parents. In fact, I was forced to become independent early on, so much so that my mother complained about it and called me "Independent Ike" (Eisenhower). But, there was a downside, since I also became needy for the love and affection that was denied to me as a baby, and I developed a deep fear of abandonment. (This was recently exemplified in my life, when my fiancé moved out after a minor argument. I ran after her, apologized, and promised to change everything about myself. In retrospect, I believe she over-reacted and she should have apologized to me).

Shortly after I was taken back home I found out that I had an older brother, Ted, whom I had never met. Ted was not united with the family until a short time after me. He had also been in a foster home. The day he came home was a momentous occasion. For awhile I thought it was normal for a brother to suddenly appear. I thought everyone was given an older brother at age 4. It was terrific to have another sibling around. He was actually a half brother but it did not make any difference in our relationship. We were as close as two brothers could be. We always shared a bedroom, which was barely big enough for one person. He had his ¾ of the room and I had my ¼. We even engaged in all the fighting that is expected of two brothers. I especially liked hanging around with him and his friends since they were five years older and appeared to be very worldly, especially about girls. As it turned out, I taught them everything they needed to know.

Ted was gifted with a terrific singing voice, which he inherited from his father. He was so talented that at age ten he was hired by the top Synagogue to sing in the choir on the high holy days. I would often sit in the front row, trying to distract him by making all kinds of stupid faces, and I would try to get him to laugh so he would not be able to sing. It never worked; he was very focused. Ted was my best friend growing up and I must give him credit for helping me excel in sports. He was an excellent athlete and taught me everything he knew, and since he was five years older, there was a lot I could learn. The most important thing in the life of a young boy, was sports. We lived for playing ball and watching the pros play, especially Mickey Mantle. For a long time I wanted to become a professional baseball player just like Mickey, who was the greatest. He was handsome, strong, muscular, fast, and humble. Despite all his injuries he was still "the best in the game". It is reported that he hit the longest home run on record, 565 feet. He was everyone's hero. Only later when he was dying from liver cancer did the fact that he was an alcoholic and womanizer come to the surface. In Mickey's final words, just before he died, he said not to use him as a role model. He was the epitome of humility and a truly great man.

In the late fifties my life had became relatively normal. The country was mellow, healing from the wounds of a World War, and for the Jews, the tragedy of the Holocaust. The entire planet needed a decade of calm and reflection. Unfortunately this would soon end in the mid-sixties, a time of great unrest and turmoil.

When I entered kindergarten my mother had me bussed many miles to a school that had an all day session instead of the half days that was offered by the school one block away. At the school we were all forced to take naps in the middle of the day. The teachers thought we were tired after running around a lot, but I think they were the ones who needed a break. It was here that I realized I must have insomnia because it was impossible for me to fall asleep during naptime. I think the other kids were also faking it. We had no choice.

While lying down, I had nothing to do except daydream. There was a tag on my blanket with what I assumed was my name. I did not know the alphabet yet, but I asked myself what other words would be sewn onto my blanket except for my name. A short time later, I was visiting my Aunt Ruth who asked me if I knew how to write my name. I had no training in writing letters and was surprised that my aunt did not know that. I proceeded to write the two words that I had looked at so many times on my blanket and indeed it was my name. My aunt was not as impressed as I thought she would be, but I impressed myself and that was enough. I realized right then that I was a genius. Too bad nobody else knew it.

I pleaded with my mother to let me go to the school that was one block away so that I could make friends with the other kids on my block. Up until now they looked at me like I was a stranger. She finally gave in and I soon became an official member of the community. It was in kindergarten that I once again experienced my attraction for the opposite sex. This time a beautiful brunette named Harriet caught my eye. I could not take my eyes off of her. Finally, I went over to her and kissed her on the lips. She did not turn away or scream so I guess she liked it. We became a couple from that day on. We kissed and held hands everyday. It was love. I had something to look forward to at school everyday. The relationship actually lasted several months. I guess I was not your average five year-old, because at that age, little boys and girls were enemies. The attraction thing is supposed to start at puberty but I had no control over my sexual urges. Little girls were so cute and bouncy.

The kissing thing really got out of hand in the second grade when I decided that I wanted to kiss every girl in the class. I would go over to girls and plant a big kiss right on their tiny, little lips. Not one of them moved away from me. I continued the kissing for several days until I realized that I should be more selective and only kiss the pretty ones. This continued for a short time until I got bored and decided to stop. Now that they were used to it they did not want to stop and came over to me for their daily smooch. I finally had to say, "no more kisses" and put an end to the whole thing. But it was great fun while it lasted.

My second love affair occurred at age seven with a gorgeous little girl named Cheryl, who lived in the apartment above mine. She was a cute and sexy blond whom I could not resist. One night my parents went out and I was told to go to her apartment so that her parents could baby-sit. When it was time to go to sleep her parents decided that we should sleep together in the same bed. Even at age 7 I knew instinctively that this was a no-no, but I certainly did not object. I also knew that I was supposed to do something to Cheryl but I did not know what it was and neither did she. Here was a golden opportunity handed to me on a silver platter and I blew it. I would never live it down. If I only knew then what I know now!

My first experience as a doctor occurred with Cheryl. We played show and tell with our anatomic differences and took make believe photos with the Brownie-Hawkeye box camera for our make believe textbook. I was very interested in documenting my findings. Too bad there was no film in the camera, but from that time on I knew I wanted to continue playing the doctor game.

The next time I manifested my interest in medicine was in the second grade, when the teacher asked all the students to draw a picture representing their favorite TV show. Most of the students depicted cartoon characters or something from the Howdy-Doody show. I, on the other hand, drew a picture of a patient on a stretcher being wheeled into the operating room from the show called "Medic", the first medical show on T. V. The teacher was so amused by my drawing that she showed it to the teacher in the next classroom. They both had a good chuckle. I didn't see the humor in it since to me it was a serious picture, but I realized that I must be different from the other students. I taught myself long division and multiplication while the class was learning simple arithmetic. I brought samples of my calculations for the teacher to review and of course she was very impressed and gave me other difficult math problems to solve. I realized that my math abilities were far more developed than my peers were. I was a smarty-pants. My self-confidence increased enormously. Unfortunately, humility lagged far behind. In spite of that I have always tried to be fair and help other people who were in need. For instance, I helped other students with their homework and gave them answers on tests. Not to brag but I was also talented in all the sports that were popular at the time such as stickball, handball, and punch ball. I was always chosen as captain of the team and would purposely pick the worst players just so they would not feel left out. I believe my talents and fairness were appreciated since I was voted president of the class every year. Naturally, my self-confidence continued to grow. This solid foundation gave me the future ability to bounce back when things became ramshackle and chaotic. However, there is a fine line between having self-confidence and being arrogant. There have been numerous times when people have accused me of the latter.

My math ability really stood out in the fourth grade class with Mrs. Garberg. She would write several math problems on the blackboard at ten o'clock every morning. By the time she was finished writing the last question I had all the answers and was ready to go up to her desk in the front of the room to get my paper graded. I would be standing there looking at the other students who were still working out the answers. The fact that I was the best in the class in math was reinforced on a daily basis. My ego grew to huge proportions. The teacher actually referred to me as "Einstein". This was better than any therapist could dream of doing for their patient's confidence. I was also a down-to-earth regular guy, and was well liked by the other students, but I started having trouble with the teachers. Since I was very bright and easily bored, I frequently disrupted the class with wisecracks. In those days, cracking jokes in class was considered a high crime. Today, unless you bring a gun to class, anything goes. The teachers did not appreciate my sense of humor (although the other students did) and I would frequently get into trouble. My grades in behavior lagged far behind those in academic subjects. On my report card I would get an A in every subject followed by a big U, circled in red, for behavior. They believed I was on the road to becoming a juvenile delinquent. I thought I was just having fun. I ask you, the reader, to decide who was right.

My father, Sidney, was a self-employed jeweler working long hours at his office on 47th street, the diamond capital of N.Y. He would come home at night, eat dinner and then continue to work at a bench he set up in the small foyer and file away, finishing off dozens and dozens of gold rings. Sometimes, I watched him work. There was very little verbal communication between us. Since he worked with his hands, it is very possible that I developed my manual dexterity by simply watching him, but I am sure genetics plays an equal role. I thought he must have been making a lot of money since he worked so many hours. Unfortunately, he had difficulty parting with it. I believe I may have inherited this trait as well. We did spend quality time together on the weekends. I remember going fishing at Prospect Park where they stocked the lake every year with new fish. The bait worms could be dug up on a hill close by. I had to insert the fishhook through the length of the worm. It was squishy and disgusting--perfect for little boys like myself. Occasionally we actually caught a fish but it was usually so small it was supposed to be thrown back. I would keep it anyway. These were fun days, sitting on the freshly cutgrass, as the sun shone through the trees, relaxing and having deep kiddy conversation with my father. He was a good listener and kibitzer and I believe I inherited my sense of humor from him. Fortunately, I am very lucky not to have inherited his nose. He has a large nose with a downward hook. Mine is smaller and straight and happens to be the best feature on my face. People frequently ask me if I have had a nose job. Sometimes I say yes and show them where the plastic surgeon signed his name. Some of my other features I did inherit from my dad including my eyes, which are hazel-brown, my hair which is frizzy and receding (thanks dad!), and the shape of my face and mouth. I guess that is more than enough.

Another fun trip we would take was to the Brooklyn Museum on a Sunday afternoon. I especially liked looking at the Egyptian collection particularly the mummies. They reminded me of one of my favorite movies, starring Boris Karloff (The Mummy). Frequently there were violin concerts in the main rotunda. Initially I found them boring but after a while I started to appreciate the beautiful music. Too bad there were no rock concerts. I also enjoyed looking at the paintings, especially in the modern art collection. The seeds of art appreciation were being planted at an early age.

Back at home, my parents were having marital problems. There were frequent arguments about money and sex which usually ended when my mother screamed at the top of her lungs and threw various objects such as silverware, small jars of mustard and anything that was handy and within reach. I would run out of the house as soon as it started. It seemed like every time my parents were together, they would argue. That is why I was almost never home. I strongly believed in see no evil, hear no evil. Finally, after 15 years of non marital-bliss, they separated. I was around 10 years old. My father was more emotional than I was when the time came for him to leave. He began to cry and said he would remember me and always love me. I really didn't think he was going to forget me. I didn't know how to respond except that I would do the same. Somehow, I felt it was much better for my parents not to be together. Finally there would be peace. This tranquility did not last very long since now that my mom didn't have my father to yell at, she took her frustrations out on me. I was screamed at on a daily basis, only to be interrupted by the phone. "Saved by the phone", I frequently thought. Her conversations lasted for hours but as soon as she was off the phone, I would run out of the house as fast as I could. If it weren't so sad it would really be funny.

At the time my father left I had little reaction except for being embarrassed when I had to explain things to my friends. I did not invite them to my house because I did not want them to ask the obvious question, "Where is your father?" I was never really close to him since he was not around when I was an infant, worked a lot while I was young and then left when I was ten. I do remember that he never got angry, never yelled, and never hit me. When he left, things were not that bad. I became more independent and had plenty of freedom, especially for a 10 year-old. All my friends had to answer to their parents for every move they made. I had no boundaries, no rules and lots of time to get into trouble.

As a result of my parents' separation, I promised myself that some day, I would get married and have a big, stable family, unlike the family life I experienced. I could not wait to find the right woman and to have children. I knew that I would have to wait until I was in my twenties, which seemed like a lifetime away. During the first several years of my parent's separation my father would make frequent visits and stay over. I had false hopes that they would get back together again. But that never happened. Soon they stopped seeing each other and instead he would come around every other Sunday to take me out. Since Ted was older and not his biological son he was not included in these visitations. During this time my brother tried unsuccessfully to develop a relationship with his biological father.

My father and I would usually go to a movie and then have White Castle hamburgers for lunch. He never liked the movie unless it was a serious drama so he could be more depressed than he was already. At age 10, I was not quite into serious drama yet. These visits stopped shortly and then the only time we would get together was when I went to his office in the city. I would see him maybe once or twice a year either near my birthday or Chanukah time, so I could shake him down for money. No wonder why he tried to avoid me!

My teacher in the sixth grade, Mrs. Harwayne, despised me (the feeling was mutual). By now my rebellious and wiseguy personality was flourishing. As the smartest and most popular kid in the class I felt I could take certain liberties. Basically, I thought I was above the law, something Woody Allen would applaud. He said that highly talented and gifted persons should be allowed to live by their own rules. It was not necessary for them to abide by the same laws that applied to everyone else. If this is not elitist I don't know what is. But it sounded good to me.

All the students in the sixth grade were required to take a test to determine who would enter a special progress program (the SP) that permitted skipping the 8th grade. Despite the fact that I scored the highest in math in the entire district, which was filled with a lot of smart Jewish kids, Mrs. Harwayne threatened that she was not going to recommend me because of my poor behavior. What nerve! She decided that at the end of each day, for the rest of the semester, I was supposed to obtain a grade for my behavior. If I had one failing day she would keep me out of the program. I was on my best behavior for about one week when I decided to stop this madness. I figured if she asked me about it, I would say, "oops, I forgot". She never said a word and probably realized she had no right to threaten my academic progress. I was not going to fit into her "goody-goody" image no matter what.

However, I realized that although academic intelligence is important, emotional intelligence is even more important. The world is already filled with Mensa misfits. The ability to get people to like you, respect you, and convince them to do what you want is paramount. There is no standardized test for this quality so it cannot be measured. You might also call it charisma, you know, the adjective attached to the late President Kennedy. Having both types of intelligence is the formula for prosperity. The key to success is sincerity and once you can fake that, you've got it made. Since I had the grades and was voted class president year after year, it appeared that I had both qualities. My only downfall was my independent and rebellious attitude, which angered some of my teachers and others in positions of authority.

I had another encounter with Mrs. Harwayne, which I am very proud of and will never forget. I was appointed to the school crossing guard the previous year, which meant I would automatically become the Captain of the squad the following year. It was quite an honor; you wore a special uniform and badge, and gave orders to the other guards. When it came time to appoint the Captain she decided to appoint someone else. In those days it was unheard of to question a teacher's authority, but I felt extremely insulted about her decision and confronted her. I told her that I was quitting the guard. She said I had a bad attitude and she would put a black mark on my permanent record. I stuck to my guns and was not going to be intimidated by her. At the time, I knew I was right and in retrospect I should have strangled her. She was wrong not to appoint me, and doubly wrong to try to intimidate a 10 year-old with her idle threats.

While growing up I used to hang out at the local grocery store. It was a way of making money since they needed somebody to deliver grocery orders in the neighborhood. I usually received between 10 cents and 25 cents depending on the order and the generosity of the deliveree. It was great to have spare change in my pocket to buy candy or comic books. I became financially independent and fiscally responsible at an early age. One day I delivered a box of groceries to the apartment of a young man. This was very unusual since all my other clients were middle aged and older women. I really did not care whom I delivered to as long as I received a nice tip. (Although anyone would agree that this man was capable of carrying his own packages). When I arrived at his apartment he was standing in front of me jingling change in his pocket and said he could not afford to give me a tip. He must have been a nut, but he was the only person ever not to give me a tip. I felt used and angry, but I vowed one day I would get my revenge. Several weeks later I was asked to deliver groceries to the same apartment. Revenge is so sweet. After I left the store, I took out the grapefruits he ordered and threw them against the wall so they would split. Next, I put the box on the floor and relieved myself all over his food. I know this was not a very nice thing to do but I was a kid and I felt he deserved it. The big question in my mind was, maybe he was going to give me an extra large tip to make up for the other day. I was playing the odds that he would not be so kind. I rang his bell and he opened his door. Again, he was standing in front of me jingling the change in his pocket, and said he did not have any money for a tip. This time, I had the last laugh. What a cheap, dirtbag! When I arrived back to the store the owner asked me if anything happened to the grapefruits. Apparently, this guy had called the store to complain. I looked at the owner quixotically, played dumb and said "I don't know", while shrugging my shoulders. I was never asked to deliver to the dirtbag again. Don't mess with me!

With the money I made as a deliveryboy, I invested in stocks and shortly thereafter I became a multimillionaire. Not! That would have been terrific, but I knew nothing about investing. At the time the adults around me did know a great deal about betting on horses though and tried to show me the scientific method they used. I asked myself, if it was so fool proof, why were they still poor schnooks living in this low-class neighborhood? I avoided the betting scheme. My hard-earned money was too valuable to lose, and the work ethic was too well ingrained at this point.

For a short time, I worked in a tiny family-run lamp factory. It was fun putting together the lamps and I thought I was doing a good job. I even showed the owner a better way to install the lamp wiring. He did not appreciate my suggestions especially since they came from a snot-nose eleven-year old. After working there for several weeks, I decided to take a twenty-minute lunch break. I thought everybody was entitled to a lunch break. I was fired immediately when I returned. I was glad to be fired because he had a retarded son working there that gave me the heebie-jeebies.

In 1960, I entered junior high school—the high point of my life. I felt like I was the smartest, best looking, most popular and most athletic boy ever. Maybe I was and maybe I wasn't, but if I had a choice to come back and remain at a certain age my entire life, I would definitely pick age 13. I am frequently told that my mental development has not progressed beyond that age. No problem! Those were the days before pimples, when I could pick and choose any girl I wanted. That is when Linda came into the picture. She was very cute and smart too. On hot summer nights we had the longest make-out sessions on record. I had to perfect the art of kissing because in those days, sex ended right there. What really intensified the relationship was that she was moving out of the neighborhood in several months time. The days before she moved were some of the saddest days. We both shed many tears because we were in love but knew it was going to end and we would probably never see each other again.

Several years later, by sheer coincidence (Kabbala please explain this one), I bumped into her at the beach. She looked similar to what I remembered only her features were more exaggerated. Her nose and chin had become longer. She lost the cuteness that she had when her features were small. She had the face of an adult but was only 16. I am sure she was still a very nice person and a great kisser, but I was no longer attracted to her. We both acted friendly wished each other well and went our separate ways. How sad! She was somebody who I thought I truly loved and yet now she was like a stranger. The Kabbala also says that love doesn't die and it is "stronger than death", but it was not so in this case. Maybe what I thought was love was really lust. I wonder what Linda thought about me.

When I turned 14, it was a great day for me because I could file for working papers and become a Good Humor boy. I waited years for this opportunity. Now I would make some real money, 5 cents for every ice cream pop. "You better be careful what you wish for because you might just get it"! I had to carry two heavy boxes filled with ice cream and dry ice on my shoulders during the hottest days of the summer, walking the entire length of the beach. I also had to scream out the words "ice cream" at the top of my lungs, continuously for eight hours every day. This job was definitely not designed for somebody who was going to become rich and famous some day. I ended up making about five dollars a day, which was not too shabby but still not worth all the work. The only fringe benefit was that I got to meet lots of hot babes in bikini bathing suits. Making money and hitting on hot babes was a workable concept but it only lasted for one summer.

In the fall I changed careers and started selling something more lightweight and manageable: pens. The plastic Bic pen had just come out and there happened to a distributor on the next block. I could buy a box of 100 pens for 5 cents each. These pens revolutionized the industry since up until now the least expensive ballpoint pens were close to a dollar. Bic was able to produce a decent product for a much better price and I was there to capitalize on it. I knew I could sell them for more than twice the price I paid. The big question was, where? I needed a place where I could find a large number of people sitting around. After not very extensive deliberations, I decided on two great areas: the subway train, and the local cafeteria. The only problem with the subway was that competition was fierce, namely the blind and severely disabled. Fortunately, I did not fit into either category and felt guilty taking business away from them. Another factor was what if I bumped into someone who knew me? Actually it did happen. One of my high school teachers saw me and asked why I was selling pens on the subway. I came up with a great answer. I told her, "I was pledging a fraternity and this was one of the tasks assigned to me". She bought the story and bought some pens.

I used to sell one pen for 15 cents and 2 for a quarter and I was constantly asked to prove that the pen could write. I found out that on the first try the pen did not write because the ink had to wet the ball. Before I went out to sell, I made sure each pen was ready to write instantly.

Another great place to sell was at Garfields Cafeteria, There were always hundreds of people sitting around the tables shooting the breeze and drinking coffee or the free seltzer, which was available to all patrons. I had my sales pitch ready: "get your wholesale pens"; they can write "over butter" and "underwater". I went over to each table with my pitch and since I was a cute kid, the adults wanted to chat with me. In order to keep me at the table they would usually buy a pen and if I made a sale at one table, the next table also wanted to buy. Occasionally the manager would come over to me and tell me to leave. I simply offered him a free pen and he would walk away very happy. I learned to be a businessman at an early age and that bribery added grease to the wheels. In several hours I would take home about 30 dollars. I retired after several months and bought a condo in Boca.

CHAPTER 2: HIGH SCHOOL AND COLLEGE

While growing up in Crown Heights, Brooklyn, we lived in a small, dark, dingy apartment that never received any sunshine and faced into an alleyway. My mom, for good reason, wanted to move. When my father lived with us they frequently went apartment hunting for a better place to live but never found it. Finally after my father moved out we decided to move to a high rise apartment complex called Trump Village in Brighton Beach. Don't get fooled by the fancy name. This was a lower middle class complex subsidized by the state and built by Fred Trump, Donald's father. There was absolutely nothing luxurious about the apartment but it was brand, spanking new and gave us an opportunity to start over. All the Jews that were being pushed out of neighborhoods in Brooklyn by the influx of Afro-Americans, decided that this was their golden opportunity to flee the old and begin anew. I felt very positive about the move since my neighborhood was deteriorating rapidly. The only problem was that I was a junior in high school and had many friends that I knew I would lose if I moved. This is a teenager's worst nightmare: to have to develop an entirely new social life that takes years to build, however getting out of the old neighborhood took precedence over my old friends who I had outgrown anyway. We had an apartment on the 20th floor that had a fabulous view, with lots of sunshine and the building was walking distance from a great beach, the world renowned, Coney Island.

As a symbolic gesture, on the day we moved in I did something that was dangerous, and which I am not proud, to this day. We owned an old, and at least in my opinion, dilapidated, bookcase. I absolutely hated this piece of furniture because it was old and it reminded me of the past. I took the bookcase, opened the window on the 20th floor, and threw it out. I watched it float in the air and fall to the ground with a loud splat. Luckily there was nobody walking in the area, otherwise they would have been crushed and I would currently be in jail for murder. It was goodbye to the old, hello to the new and in a perverse way, I felt good about what I had done. It was a purging experience but I think I must have been temporarily insane. Without my knowing, it might have been a valuable antique, but at the time I could not tell what an antique was if it hit me over the head (no pun intended).

Although this act did not send me to jail, I have had several scrapes with the law where I did end up in the slammer. I am not proud of these incidents but they are part of my life story and did play a role in shaping my character. Although each of these experiences was very traumatic at the time, when viewed in perspective, they at least provide a few chuckles.

The first incident occurred when I was 15 and had just moved into Trump Village. There was a party for teenagers in one of the six buildings in the area. It was an excellent way to meet new people and pick up babes. I thought, maybe at this shindig I would get lucky. My best friend Richie and I tried to enter the party but were immediately turned away by the security guard at the door because we did not live in that building. I tried to reason with him and told him that the party was for anyone who lived in Trump but he still refused to let us in. I knew I was right and decided to enter anyway. As he attempted to push me away, I put up my hands to protect myself and accidentally pushed his thumb backwards. Immediately he yelled out that I had broken his thumb and accused me of assaulting him when in fact I was just trying to protect myself. He called his superiors who then called the police and before you can say "supercallafragalisticexpialladoshus", I was arrested and on my way to jail. Richie stood by me as a loyal friend and was arrested as well. This incident reinforced my belief that I was living in a corrupt society where right is wrong and vice-versa. Why should I be arrested when the security guard was the one who did the assaulting? He should have been arrested. It seemed that reason and intelligence took a backseat to power and authority, just like in a dictatorship. We were released later that night but the party was already over. Afterwards, we were considered heroes by our peers for being rebels and bucking the establishment.

I had to appear in court several weeks later where I was assigned a public defender that did not even want to hear my side of the story. He was one of the most rude and impatient people I had ever met up until that time. My defense was that I was a grade A student, therefore a good kid, and this incident was a big mistake. We showed my report card to the judge who quickly glanced at it, never once looked at me, and quickly dismissed the case. Justice finally prevailed. I learned that if I did well in school I could get away with almost anything.

I look back at high school with fond memories but there were two major pressures on every one of us. One was academic pressure: getting good grade and doing extra-curricular activities that would help get you into a good college. The other was peer pressure to look cool and hang out with a cool crowd. Luckily, I did well at both. Academically, I excelled in math and science and did above average in English and social studies. I always found math to be a challenge and believed it to be very important in the scheme of things. I thought English was a bullshit subject for girls and sissies. Little did I know that it is much more important to communicate than to add a bunch of numbers. Socially, I was popular, had many friends, and never had a problem attracting the opposite sex. As a matter of fact I came in second place in a popularity contest in the ninth grade. My life was "peachy keen" but I cannot say the same for my skin, which soon became "creatures and cream", due to a severe case of acne. During breakouts I was so embarrassed that I sometimes did not go to school. Too bad I didn't have stock in Clearasil at the time. I tried every remedy known to mankind and even went as far as getting radiation treatments, which had dangerous side effects, but did the trick. I eventually went for skin peelings to remove the pockmarks. An extremely painful acid was applied to my face in order to burn the top layers of skin which would eventually peel off, leaving nice pink skin from the underneath layers. I learned early on that it was often necessary to endure pain in order to achieve beauty.

Among the many incidents that had occurred up until now, there was one major event that could have had been devastating. I was taking a mid term exam and had a "jip" sheet among the exam papers on my desk. I was famous for having the best "jip" sheets in the school since I was able to copy the entire year's information of any one course on a tiny piece of paper in the smallest of print. I was very proud of this accomplishment and even thought about selling the sheets to others. Just the making of the sheet was a challenge and education. While I was helping a friend who was sitting next to me during the exam, the teacher walked past my desk and spotted the sheet. He quickly removed all the papers on my desk, asked me to leave the room, and reported me for cheating. I was immediately suspended for two days, required to sit in the guidance counselor's office and do nothing except lament my situation. I was embarrassed but not terribly upset by the whole experience. Why not? I knew it would pass after a few days and then things would go back to normal. A recent survey of high school students indicated that eighty per-cent cheat on exams, so I guess I was in good company. But I believe I was very lucky that the school did not make a bigger deal about it. Afterall, I could have been expelled and then would have had a lot of explaining to do when it came time to apply to college.

It was around this time that I was beginning to think seriously about what I wanted to be when I grew up. I never had a desire to become a fireman or policeman like most kids. My decision to go into medicine was influenced by watching a very popular movie that had just come out about the life of a doctor. It depicted the doctor as a great man, handsome, cool and dedicated to saving lives. He was a God-like figure who was revered by all, was extremely over-worked, and who sacrifices his personal life to save mankind. What a romantic notion! The most impressive part of the movie was that he is constantly sought after by beautiful women, who would throw themselves at him and who want to be his wife. The image in the movie was a sharp contrast to my family doctor who was a bald, rotund man with a disgusting cigar hanging out of his mouth dripping with saliva. His usual advice was to watch your diet and not to smoke. I guess he was following the "hypocritic oath" instead of the "Hippocratic Oath". He died in his fifties, the average life expectancy of G. P.s at the time. Despite the way he looked, his intelligence and compassion did leave me with a permanent positive image of what a doctor is supposed to be like. I wanted to be just like him minus the cigar, the fat, and the saliva.

Another significant influence on my decision to become a doctor was as a result of an injury that I sustained, while jumping down a flight of steps at age fourteen. I twisted my knee and felt a sudden onset of severe pain worse than I had ever felt before. Usually pain lasts for several minutes and then goes away. This pain lasted for hours. I knew there was a seriously problem right away as I limped home, hopping on one leg. When the pain finally dissipated and I was able to move my knee I felt a loose piece of bone popping in and out of the joint. It floated around to different parts of my knee and sometimes I could feel it right under my skin. I could not run or participate in any sports. Off to the doctors! This is when I was first introduced to orthopedics. We made an appointment with two of them in Brooklyn, a young one who had no bedside manner and who had a argument with my mother; and an old one who appeared to me to be senile. My mother insisted upon second and third opinions way before they were popular. To her credit, I finally ended up with the top orthopedist in the country, the chief at The Joint Disease Hospital of N.Y. He put me in a cast for a short period but the floating bone kept popping out of place so surgery appeared to be the only answer. My dream of becoming a professional baseball player began to evaporate. At that time there was very little money to be made in baseball so I was not too upset. Little did I know that that would soon change. I sometimes wonder what my life would have been like if I had taken that route. Another reason I did not pursue baseball was that it was not a Jewish thing to do. Good Jewish boys became doctors, lawyers and accountants, not baseball players. We were encouraged to use our minds not our hands. There were very few Jewish athletic role models outside of Hank Greenberg and Sandy Koufax. Since Greenberg was popular in the forties, which was before I was born, I did not identify with him. Koufax was truly heroic and not only was he one of the greatest pitcher of our time, he will go down in the annals of Jewish sports history for refusing to pitch in a World Series game because it was Yom Kippur. If I was being paid as much as he was, I seriously doubt I would have refused. I would tell the chief of Rabbis to try to move the holiday to a different day. Let's not be coy, we all know that money is the most important factor in a Jewish person's life. It's a genetic thing; we can't do anything about it. Koufax was great but every Jewish and non-Jewish boy alike wanted to be just like Mickey Mantle, not Sandy Koufax. Hitting was always more important than pitching. Also, let's not forget that to a Brooklyn boy, the Dodgers (Koufax' team) were traitors when they moved to L. A.

After putting my sports life on hold for about two years and walking with a limp (hence the nickname-peg-leg), I finally consented to surgery and was admitted into the hospital. I should have had surgery much earlier but it was considered verboten at the time. I felt very macho that I was going for surgery. The operation involved cutting open my knee and removing four pieces of loose bone and cartilage that had broken off into the knee joint. Just before the procedure, while in the O.R. holding room, the surgeon who was 75 years old, asked me how I was doing. I was doing fine until he came over. As he was talking his hands were shaking like a leaf. Uh oh! Maybe I could change my mind before it was too late. In the end, since I had psyched myself up for the surgery, I decided to go ahead anyway. If I knew I would have to endure such severe pain right after the operation, I definitely would have cancelled. Each time I woke up, I pleaded for more morphine, not just for the pain, but to knock me out. I slept for almost three days before I started feeling better and I was in the hospital for a total of three weeks. Today, I would have been kicked out after two days.

While I was a patient in the hospital, I decided that I was going to become a doctor. Why? Because of a pretty girl of course! She was in a bed in the next room also recovering from surgery on her leg. She was seventeen, two years older than me, and seemed so intelligent and wise. We talked for hours about everything. One day we were in the middle of a conversation when her doctor walked in. He looked like the archetypal nerd, i.e. thick glasses, red hair and freckles, a lab coat with a pencil holder in the breast pocket, and absolutely no personality. He spoke like he had taken speech lessons from Elmer Fudd. In spite of all this, when he walked into the room, she interrupted our conversation and turned away from me like I did not exist. I walked out of her room unnoticed and a light turned on in my head. If I became a doctor I would get the attention of women no matter how geeky I looked and no matter how nerdy I became. Just imagine if I was a doctor and stayed somewhat cool at the same time. The possibilities were endless. From then on my goals were set in stone. The money and prestige was fine but the chance to become a babe magnet was the key. Helping people and excelling in science are the reasons I gave publicly but privately I knew the real reason.

The surgery on my knee was successful and once again I was able to participate in all sports several months later. The only evidence that I had undergone surgery was the huge scar that extends across my entire knee joint. The girl I met in the hospital did call me several times after I was discharged but we did not meet again. Good luck wherever you are and thank you for unknowingly helping me make my career choice.

Another important factor in my decision to become a doctor was financial security. I grew up living a lower middle class life style and was envious of my friends whose families obviously had more money than mine did. That doesn't mean I did not have adequate food or shelter but did not have the luxuries that other people had. I became a "material boy" way before Madonna, except for a short time in college, when I renounced capitalism and became a hippie. Aside for that short period of time, I felt deprived and wanted all the luxuries that I did not have while growing up. By becoming a doctor I was guaranteed to have an opulent lifestyle.

After I moved to Trump, I transferred in my senior year to Lincoln High and decided to get the hell out of school early by doubling up on bull-shit English classes. This would allow me to graduate in January instead of June and gave me a six-month hiatus from academia. It was a smart move. After-all, I was going to spend the next decade in school

For the next six months I built up a successful business as a carpenter and handyman. There was a dire need for my services at Trump Village since every new apartment needed work. Initially, I invested fifty dollars to print business cards and buy a power drill and saw. This was a significant investment for me, but I was confident that my business would thrive, and it did. One of the most frequent requests was the shaving off the bottom of doors. Since the floors were not wood every tenant installed carpet through-out the apartment. Invariably the doors between the rooms would not be able to open or close. That's where I came in. I would remove the door from the hinge and using a circular saw I cut off one inch from the bottom of the door. The maintenance men were charging 5 dollars per door. I knew it would take about 5 minutes to do the job so I could charge half the price and still make out well. Each apartment had about 6 doors to shave. It would take less than an hour including schmoozing with the tenant and I could make fifteen bucks which at today's prices, is about 75 dollars per hour, cash. There were also other types of jobs such as installing extra locks on the inside of the front door (everybody was very paranoid about robberies and had three or four locks), hanging lighting fixtures, hanging traverse rods for drapes and curtains etc. I was in such demand that I hired a friend of mine, Gary, to help. I was rolling in dough and questioned whether I should go to college or continue my business. Sanity prevailed and my dream of becom-ing a doctor was not sidetracked by my newfound riches. However, the ex-perience I obtained as a carpenter was invaluable and helped me become a better orthopod and businessman.

At the time, my best friend Gary was planning to go to Merchant Marine academy and encouraged me to get a job working on a ship. The pay was excellent and you were able to travel and see the world. As a teenager this idea was very romantic and exciting. But in order to get a job on a ship you had to have Seaman's papers, and in order to get Seaman's papers you needed to have a promise of a job. This was my first real life Catch-22. Gary gave me the bright idea of telling them that I was in the Merchant Marine Academy, was on my summer break and wanted to ship out. They would surely be sympathetic. I pulled it off, got my papers, and quickly got a job as an engineer on a freighter carrying cars (probably stolen) from N.Y. to Puerto Rico. It was great! I slept in the officers quarters and was fed what to me at the time was gourmet food. Shortly into the trip, which was one week, I realized what scoundrels and drunks these men really were. Everybody hated each other and was ready to stab each other in the back. One day I accidentally locked myself out of my room, and didn't know what to do because I was too embarrassed to tell anybody. My neighbor next door seemed like a nice person so I asked his advice. He suggested that I go out of his porthole window and swing my arm over to my porthole window, pull myself up and climb through. Since I trusted this guy it sounded like a good idea. Like a complete and total idiot I proceed to climb through his window. As I am hanging from his porthole with my body pressed against the side of the ship, about 20 feet above the water, I realized that if I my hands slip I am a dead man. I also realized that my "friend" fooled me and didn't care if I lived or died. I said a prayer and with the help of God, I swung my hand and body to my window, climbed in, and of course didn't speak to that ass-hole for the rest of the trip. The drunken bastard is probably still laughing about the whole thing.

As a senior in high school I did what every smart Jewish boy did and applied to Brooklyn College. It was considered an excellent school in those days, before they started the open admissions policy. Getting into Brooklyn College was a significant achievement since they only admitted the smartest kids. After having been accepted, I went there for orientation. That was enough to convince me not to stay. I was surrounded by the largest collection of nerdy, pencil-necked geeks I had ever seen in one room. No way was I going to spend the next four years with these guys. No freakin' way! I was made for much bigger and better things and if I stayed I might end up looking and acting like them. Another factor was that I absolutely did not want to live at home while going to college. My college aspirations were not high since I could not pay for the likes of Harvard or Yale so I applied to the poor mans Harvard, Harpur College (SUNY-Binghamton). This was the best state school and had a terrific reputation. It is still considered one of the top state schools in the country.

Just before going off to college was the perfect time to make changes in the way I looked. I always envied the jet-black straight hair look. Unfortunately, I was blessed with brown brillo-hair. First, I dyed my hair black and then I straightened it. I entered college with my new improved cool look. Little did I know this new look would rapidly change. The black hair reacted to the sun by turning red, at the same time that the new hair was growing in brown, and the straight hair was being replaced by the brillo. I ended up with straight and kinky, black, red and brown, hair. Nobody could figure what was happening on the top of my head. It definitely was unique just like my personality. I now know why I fit in so well with the offbeat, on the edge type of person. Of course my unusual hairdo was an outgrowth of my wild personality not vise-versa. I enjoyed experimenting, living on the edge and taking chances. I believed in experiencing as much as possible. Helen Keller once said "a life without risk is not worth living'. Along with taking risks, three passions governed my life: the longing for love, the search for knowledge, and the quest for power.

I started Harpur College during the summer semester of July 1965 when there were a total of 300 students. It felt more like a summer camp than a college. Because I had street smarts and an outgoing personality I soon was catapulted to chief counselor. Being away from home, equipped with a newfound freedom, I sought out danger and left behind a litany of stories that were no doubt recorded in the oral history of the college. For instance, one night I sneaked into the girls' dormitory, climbed on the roof and removed the flag, a pink bunny rabbit, which was on the top of the dorm, replacing it with a flag of skull and crossbones. It was the talk of the campus for the next few days until the maintenance men took it down. Next, I masterminded a plot to break into the student center in the middle of the night and steal all of the fraternity plaques off the walls. Six of us were involved and each had a specific job assigned. It was as close as you can get to a Hollywood movie bank heist except there were no cameras. It was executed with the precision of a Swiss watch. And again, it was the talk of the campus. We published a list of demands that each fraternity had to comply with if they wanted their plaques to be returned. One of the demands involved having the brother's walk around the campus naked. Unfortunately, they drew the line at nudity. After several weeks we decided to break in again and put the plaques back.

One night while eating dinner in the cafeteria I watched a delivery of huge bags of chopped meat being brought into the kitchen and decided we should have "hamburger night" at the dorm. I brazenly walked into the kitchen and walked out with a bag of meat in front of everybody and not a word was said. Later that night all of us had burgers, which tasted especially good since they were free.

One of the most notorious pranks occurred when I enacted a mock murder of a fellow student in order to get a reaction out of our very complacent dorm counselor, Neil. The other student and myself started yelling at each other in front of the closed door of Neil's room. I screamed, "I am going to kill you", applied ketchup onto his shirt, and lit a firecracker. He fell down and played dead while I ran away. Neil bolted out of his room, looked at the bloody dead body in front of his door, and proceeded to call the police. It took three of us to pull the phone out of his hands and convince him it was just a prank.

The first year of college was an experiment in freedom for me since I was on my own and did not have to answer to anybody except myself. I was not concerned about getting good grades; instead I was interested in getting bad girls. After receiving a "C" average I knew I would have to change my attitude if I were going to have any chance of becoming a doctor. I was competing against the smartest students in the school who unlike myself had one goal in mind: getting into med school which was an extremely difficult task.

During my second semester at Harpur I attended a very popular beer blast called Paddy's wake. Once upon a time there was a very conscientious student named Paddy who always ran to the library right after dinner to get the best seat. It was a typical winter night in Binghamton with many patches of ice dotting the campus. While running and holding his pencil in his hand he accidentally slipped on the ice and fell forward onto his pencil, which pierced his chest, and went into his heart, killing him instantly. Every year the college commemorates this tragedy with a party. I am not sure this story is true but any excuse for a party is a good one by me.

Barbara was standing alone looking real cool, very pretty and petite, wearing sexy, tight, blue jeans, a tight sweater, and smoking a cigarette. It was late in the evening, I hadn't found anybody special, and I was looking for someone to dance with. There she was Barbara Backer, in the right place at the right time. I went over to her in my cocky and confident manner, ready to get rejected, and asked her to dance. I was astonished when she said yes and could not figure out why a woman of such beauty would answer in the affirmative until we began to dance. She danced like Elaine on "Seinfeld", off the beat and uncoordinated. This actually intrigued me. She was the picture of cool and yet had a hidden, vulnerable side. I asked to be excused to go to the men's room and told her to wait. This was a ploy to see if the other person was truly interested. When I came back she was still there in the same spot waiting for me as I requested. I knew I was in, for better or worse. I asked her if she wanted a beer and she said "yes". It is always good to get them a little drunk and then make the big move. The beer was waiting under my coat. I did not want to wait on a big line so when I arrived at the party I went right over to the beer line while nobody was waiting. She was very impressed by this well thought out move. I, in turn was impressed by her when she whipped out a pack of Pall-Mall unfiltered cigarettes. These were one of the strongest brands especially when compared to my wimpy Kent filters. When she tried to light the cigarette, I learned a lot about who she was. She did not know how to properly light the match or the cigarette. I laughed to myself. The cool image she was trying to display was as transparent as the cellophane around the pack of cigarettes. But it was charming. The relationship was sealed when we were ready to leave and she put on her coat. It was a brown pea coat. This was the coolest and most stylish coat one could wear.

A blue pea coat was cool but a brown one was a notch above. I took her home and kissed her goodnight; she was an excellent kisser.

Barbara told me she was an 18 year old, sophomore and asked for my stats. At the time I was a 17-year-old, freshman. I knew that I could not reveal this to her for fear of being immediately rejected, so I told her I was 20, a junior, and transferred from another school. She bought it! Nine months later I was driving in the city with Barbara and was stopped by the police for a traffic violation. The cop looked at my license and asked out-loud "Are you 18"? I answered very quietly in the affirmative while I looked over to Barbara to see if she was listening. The cop let me off but she didn't. "How dare you lie to me. I never want to see you again!" was what I heard next. I begged and pleaded and tried to explain that she would not have gone out with me if I told her the truth right away. This was our first big fight. I persisted with my apology over and over, day after day. I appealed to the fact that I looked and acted older than my real age. Bingo! She finally accepted my apology and we were a couple once again. Although we have had our differences, we were married 4 years later and stayed married for 24 years. Barbara and I still have a great affection, great friendship, and four great kids.

My grades in the first year of college were abysmal and I knew I better get to work or I would never have a prayer of a chance of getting into medical school. By the second year I knew I had turned the corner when I received an "A" in organic chemistry, the course that is known to separate the men from the boys. The textbook was the largest I had ever seen but I studied so hard that I was able to walk out of the final exam in half the given time and waved to my peers as I left. The next semester I did so well in physical chemistry, another killer course, that my professor exempted me from the final exam.

After my junior year, when it came time to apply to medical school, I still had a relatively low average compared to other pre-med students. The medical schools were not knocking down my door and I received numerous rejections. I had to think of possible alternative plans such as dental or osteopath school, or possibly robbing banks. When it came time to take the pre-dental exam, I overslept. I guess I really did not want to be a dentist after all. I applied to osteopath school because it was considered much easier to get accepted, although I knew nothing about the field. When it came time to take an interview with an osteopath in town, I walked into his office and was freaked out. His office was ancient. I thought I was back in the 1800's. The doctor himself looked like a member of the Barber Shop Quartet of the 1890's. My impression of osteopathy became reduced to zero. I viewed him as a quack. Not until I went into private practice and worked with other osteopaths did I realize that he was probably eccentric and that they are regular doctors just like MD's.

Next, it was suggested that I start making inquiries into foreign medical schools in such countries as Mexico, Italy, and Spain. I quickly nixed that idea when I was told that I would have to learn another language. The only subject I ever failed was a foreign language and I had enough problems with English. How could I ever learn a new language on top of the difficult medical school curriculum?

St. Louis University was still considering my application, so I decided to make a bold move by calling the dean and setting up a personal interview. This was my last chance since every other school had rejected me. The next day I flew to St. Louis where there had just been a major snowstorm and the city had come to a complete halt. I did not know that this act of God would help me clinch my place in medicine. My plane had trouble landing but finally the pilot was cleared. Luckily, I immediately found a taxi. The roads had just been plowed and were empty so I arrived at the school in plenty of time for my interview. I changed my clothes in the bathroom and put on the only suit I owned. Previously, at the airport, while waiting for my plane, I took a haircut and shave. I did not think it would be a good idea to be seen with hair down to my shoulders and a beard to match. I took my interview with the Dean of Admissions who was extremely impressed with the fact that I was able to get to the interview on time during this major snowstorm. I explained to him how important it was for me to become a doctor and that I would be one of the best, if he would only give me the opportunity. I flew back to school with my fingers crossed and a prayer on my lips. A week later, on April Fools Day, I received a letter from St. Louis. I looked at it very closely to see if it was legitimate because I thought for sure, it was a sadistic prank. I opened the letter and read the good news: I was accepted. My dream had come true. I saved the letter and framed it. Recently, I sent the school a five, thousand dollar donation, thanking them for giving me the opportunity to become a doctor.

Unfortunately, I had a most devastating encounter with the law, one month after I had been accepted into medical school. My dream of becoming a doctor was about to evaporate. During the late sixties and early seventies pot smoking was rampant on the campuses of every college. It coincided with the "make love not war", anti-establishment, anti-Vietnam, "Hippie" movement that was prevalent at the time. While I was home for the holidays, I picked up a small quantity of pot in the city with the purpose of using some and selling the rest at school. I returned to school and was approached by a friend who told me he knew people who wanted to buy my pot. He pointed out who they were. They looked a little older, not very cool, but wore the hippie attire that was popular at the time. I knew that selling pot was against the law so I devised a plan that I thought would circumvent the law. In retrospect it was one of the stupidest things I ever did. I would give the pot to my friend behind a closed door who would then give it to his friends, take money from them, and then hand the money to me behind a closed door. What a fantastic plan! Technically speaking he made the sale. Unfortunately, the plan did not work. The following week, on a Friday night, while I was having a party in my room, I heard a knock on my door. Before I could find out who it was, ten State Police, dressed in cheap black suits, barged into my room and announced that we were all under arrest. We had just smoked some excellent weed and were quite high when they walked in. For a split second it seemed like a bad dream until reality set in. I was informed that I sold pot to an undercover agent and then I was handcuffed, brought to jail, fingerprinted and photographed just like on T. V. The bust made the front page of the Binghamton Press and I was described as a drug kingpin. Finally, in the middle of the night, after many hours, I was put in a tiny cell. I just wanted to go to sleep and hopefully, when I woke up the whole thing would disappear.

I could not believe the size of the mattress they provided for me. It was about an inch thick and perfect for a small cat or dog. There was a lot of noise coming from the convicts in the other cells. Since I was a really tough guy from Brooklyn I thought I could assert myself. I shook the bars of my cell and yelled out in the meanest voice I could muster, that everybody should shut the f-ck up, because I was trying to sleep, and I would kick their ass if they didn't listen. To my amazement it become really quiet for about 5 minutes, but it didn't last. The other felons called my bluff and went back to their previous level of noise.

I was bailed out the next day and given a court date to return. While I was in jail the Dean of the college called me to see if I was O.K. and if I needed anything. Without skipping a beat I asked him to send over the books I would need to study for my upcoming chemistry test. He was extremely impressed that under the circumstances my priority was to crack the books. My request for books unknowingly helped me later.

The college felt it was their duty to inform St. Louis Medical School that I was indicted for selling pot. With that information I would have surely been rejected. What school would take a chance on a student whom had been in jail for selling drugs? None on this planet! Somehow, I had to convince the Dean not to inform St. Louis because of the expected consequence and because I was innocent until proven guilty. This time my mother came to my rescue. She explained to the Dean the unusual circumstances of my life and how I overcame many obstacles to get to where I am today. The poverty! The orphanage! The divorced parents! She also threw in the fact that she was sick, just to ram it home. The combination of her appeal to sympathy and my dedication to studying even though I was in jail, convinced the Dean not to send a report. I was given another lucky break. Fortunately, when my case reached the court my attorney convinced the judge that I was an upstanding member of the community and that the arrest was an aberration. The Judge decided to withhold any decision for 2 years to see if I got into any more trouble during that time. The fact that I was at the top of my class in medical school at the time the case was reevaluated helped sway his decision to drop the case. Another stroke of luck! Otherwise I would be writing this book from a jail cell rather than my study (notwithstanding the fact that some excellent pieces of literature have been written from behind bars).

CHAPTER 3: MEDICAL SCHOOL, MARRIAGE, & ORTHOPEDICS

My first year in medical school was an extremely difficult year for me. Apart from the academic pressures, I lived in a fraternity house in the heart of St. Louis with a group of straight-laced Midwesterners that had never been out of the cornfields and had never seen a Jew. They actually believed that Jews had horns growing out of the top of their head like the famous sculpture of Moses, by Michelangelo. With my long, kinky-fro, mustache, and muttonchops, I really stood out. It didn't matter because I was there not to make friends but to become the world's best doctor. I dreamed about finding the cure for cancer and becoming famous. I thought that the way to become a great doctor was to obtain the highest grades. Since this belief is common among medical students, competition is keen. Having just graduated from a top Northeast school with a plethora of smart, competitive students, I was way ahead of the game. I also needed to maintain excellent grades to prove to the Judge that my previous arrest was a big mistake. Lastly, I needed to prove something to myself. Sometimes I felt that I was not worthy of becoming a physician and should not have been accepted into medical school. Don't worry the feeling usually only lasted for a few seconds! I actually became one of the top students in the class.

I knew I was on the right track one month into the semester after a big biochemistry test. After the exam was graded the professor walked into the classroom, posted the dismal results, and berated the entire class for such a poor performance. The grades ranged from 15 to 85, with an average of 42. I thought I did OK, probably about a 60, but to my amazement I scored an 85, the highest in the class. I tried to show no emotion but inside I was beaming and knew there would be smooth sailing ahead.

During my first year in St. Louis I had my third brush with the law. I purchased an old jalopy, a 1954 Pontiac that I affectionately called the "yellow bomb", for $50 from a fellow student. I found an expired Florida license plate in the street and slapped it on the car. Barbara, who was attending grad school in the next state, was visiting me and we decided to take a leisurely drive through the park. It turned out not to be so leisurely since I ended up in the clinker. I accidentally sideswiped another car while I was making a turn and decided to drive away from the scene since I had no driver's license and phony plates. Trust me, driving away in this car was almost impossible since there was no acceleration. In spite of this, I was pulling away from the other car when Barbara insisted that I stop my car. I tried to explain that I could get into a lot of trouble but she didn't listen and insisted I do the right thing. In deference to her I stopped the car and just as I predicted, I got into a lot of trouble. The police were called and I was arrested for leaving the scene of an accident and driving without a license. I was going to be put in jail unless I came up with $250 bail. I only had $20 in my wallet. Since I did not know anybody in St. Louis who could put up that kind of money, I called the Dean of the medical school and asked him for help. What was I thinking? I must have been insane. He should have been the last person to call. Of course the Dean refused to bail me out but he did recommend that I call a bondsman which I did. I was then released on my own recognizance. Everybody in the school found out, but instead of being treated like a scofflaw, I actually became a minor celebrity.

My next stupid mistake occurred when I appeared in court to defend myself without an attorney. I wore my white medical school jacket with my stethoscope dangling out of the pocket and thought the judge would be sympathetic to a medical student. He probably was but stilled fined me $35, which I was unable to pay. When I explained that I did not bring any money, he ordered the sheriff to lock me up. They swiftly took me away and were about to put me behind bars when I asked if I could make a call. They granted me my wish and luckily on the first try I reached a friend who said she would bring the money right away and get me out. The sheriff was not willing to wait and continued to process me like any other criminal along with the mother-rapers and father-stabbers. I was fingerprinted and handed a striped uniform to wear when my friend finally arrived. Thirty-five dollars later the debacle was over and I was finally released.

St. Louis was a primitive town compared to the Big Apple. The anti-war, hippie movement which was pervasive in the rest of the country had yet to arrive in the Midwest. I felt that I did not fit in and needed to plan an escape. It would be impossible to leave in the first year of school, but in the second year I began to contemplate my move. It took a dare from a friend to get me really motivated. "You don't have the balls to transfer", were his exact words. I always loved a good challenge. I started the wheels rolling by sending for an application to Downstate in Brooklyn, my hometown. When I graduated college I didn't even think of applying to Downstate since it reminded me of Brooklyn College, populated by geeks and nerds. After experiencing the Midwest lifestyle I just wanted to go home to familiar territory, geeks and all.

I needed a really good excuse to transfer, so I came up with a foolproof excuse--I had a sick mother to take care of. It wasn't a complete lie since my mother was frequently sick. She had some kind of "chronic fatigue" syndrome that had no name at the time but has since become a commonly diagnosed condition. It was not enough to have a terrific excuse, one also needed to have top grades (I was third in the class) and a high score on the National Boards, a test given to medical students after the second year. I was informed by Downstate that there were only three openings and 150 applicants. The odds were heavily against me. It was more difficult to transfer schools than to get accepted into the first year. I studied my butt off for the boards and received a superior score. Then I knew I had an excellent chance. I finally did get accepted to Downstate and said goodbye to St. Louis for what I thought would be forever. To my surprise, thirty years later I returned with my son, Josh. He was starting college at one of the top schools in the country, Washington University, located in St. Louis. This is a true-life example of "what goes around comes around".

During the summer of '69, I attended a famous rock concert at Woodstock. It was five days of music, love, peace, and drugs. It brought together an entire nation of hippies and peaceniks that were previously fragmented all over the country. A half million of us gathered together in one space and we became a movement that would grow rapidly until we were the majority in most urban areas. We helped change the government policy with regard to Vietnam and led the nation towards a more spiritual and peace-loving state of mind. Let's not forget about the more pleasurable aspects of our movement, which included sexual liberation and pot smoking. The entire country, and world, went on a mind-expanding journey that permanently changed people's lifestyles.

By the following summer of 1970, Barbara (my girlfriend for 5 years) and I decided to take the plunge and get married. Basically, it was either we get married or we break up, and the former was a much more attractive choice. Although I was very much in love I waited so long just in case there was a famous movie star that desperately wanted me. No such luck! However, Barbara was beautiful and sexy and when she smiled she reminded me of a pixie. I also knew she would be a good mother and I wanted to have many kids. I dreamed of having a large and stable family life unlike the one that I had in my childhood. I despised the singles scene with its pervasive phoniness and superficiality. It would also be nice to come home to one person who cared about me, and have a hot dinner ready for me when I walked through the door. Let's not forget about having somebody to share my mattress at the end of the day. A warm body is much better than a fluffy pillow. We had a small but elegant wedding including an outdoor ceremony with flute music. At the time it was considered very avant-garde. There was plenty of dancing, drinking, and pot smoking.

Barbara proved to be an excellent wife. She had a good job as an assistant editor for a magazine and supported the two of us. She helped to keep me on a steady path so I may reach my goals, which at the time was to finish medical school and become a terrific doctor.

At this point, I was now a happily married man, not HAPPY, but happy, back on my home turf and a third year medical student. This is the year that students finally get to apply everything they have learned for the past two years and work directly with patients. They enter the hospital as doctors-wearing white coats, and with stethoscopes hanging out of their pockets. Although we were called "doctors", we felt very insecure in this newly acquired role. The nurses smirked behind our backs about our naivete, and played little power games just to put us in our place and make us feel more insecure.

Upon entering medical school, my ambition was to become a psychiatrist. With my normal zeal, I tried to read as much as possible on the subject. Why psychiatry? I believe I was trying to understand the neurotic personalities of my mother and father. One was a paranoid schizophrenic while the other was a manic-depressive. I believe the blending of these pathologies produced my unique personality! It was only after I worked as an extern (between my second and third year of school), on the psychiatric unit at Kings County Hospital did I come to my senses and change my career choice. For some strange reason I did not find anything wrong with the patients. They appeared normal to me. Instead, the doctors and nurses seemed to have serious mental problems. After one patient tried to commit suicide with a razor blade and another patient escaped from the ward did I finally realize that I had no clue about mental disease. What really ended it for me was when I took psychiatry in my third year. I believe the instructor hated me and I likewise. I was so worried that he was going to find out there was something mentally wrong with me that I became extremely self-conscious, had trouble sleeping and needed to take Valium just to sit in class. Every other student appeared relaxed while I felt like a wound-up spring ready to explode. When I barely passed the course I realized this was not for me. I needed another career path. What would it be? I decided to try a medical subspecialty.

I took an elective in Endocrinology, the study of the glands and hormones. I was placed into a one on one situation with an instructor who looked and acted like Dufus Dulecti. After two days with him I decided to move on and came to the conclusion that I did not like any area of internal medicine. This was very disconcerting since I had dedicated and sacrificed many years of my life in order to become a doctor and now that I have reached that goal I was not at all interested. I did not want to sit around pontificating about diseases and writing a myriad of prescriptions, which is what most medical doctors do. I was very skeptical about all medications because of their numerous side effects. So often medications made patients even worse. A second pill had to be prescribed to counteract the complications of the first pill, and so on. I did not accept the basic philosophy inherent in mainstream medicine. I leaned towards a more holistic approach, helping the body heal itself with minimal interference. Since I was always good with my hands, I thought perhaps I should pursue a career in surgery. However, I also felt that there was too much unnecessary surgery being performed. I promised myself that I would be different and perform an operation only when it was absolutely necessary. I might starve but I was going to stay true to my beliefs.

One of the areas of medicine that I did not learn anything about while in medical school was taking care of injuries such as strains sprains broken bones, etc. How was I supposed to be a well-rounded doctor without knowing anything about these basic concepts? I decided to take orthopedics (the branch of medicine concerned with bone and joint injuries and diseases) and as luck would have it, there was an immediate opening. This was not a particularly popular elective at the time because mixed in with the more interesting cases were the patients with chronic diseases such as polio and bone infections. These patients had long-standing problems that were frequently incurable. Some of these patients stayed in the hospital for many months at a time. The doctor was repeatedly faced with a sense of failure. It is always preferable to be able to treat a condition and send the patient home in a few days, completely cured. At that time only about one half of the patients fit into the fast cure category. However, things have changed dramatically since then. The vast majority of patients do obtain a fast cure while chronic patients have almost disappeared from the scene as new high tech procedures have been introduced. Total joint replacements with high-density plastics and arthroscopic laser surgery are just a few examples. Now, orthopedics has become one of the most desired specialties and only the top students are offered a position.

The first day as a student in orthopedics I met the other residents and instantly felt a connection. They were regular guys interested in sports, spoke in a casual down-to-earth manner, and were a different breed of doctor. On the second day, I was given the opportunity to operate on a fractured hip. This was one of the most common procedures that an orthopedist had to treat and would usually take about 3-4 hours to complete. The fractured bones had to be put back together with a plate and screws to hold it in place. It was similar to the carpentry that I had done as a teenager and mechanical engineering for which I had a natural talent. Even though it was my first time, I finished the procedure in less than half the normal time and did a great job. The chief resident who was monitoring me was amazed and called it beginner's luck, but I knew he was wrong. That night I went home feeling great, told Barbara about the surgery, opened up a bottle of champagne, and celebrated. I found my calling! I was going to be an orthopedic surgeon and a great one at that! I didn't care how much money I made (I was not going to starve), and I didn't care that we were not considered the intellectuals of the medical community. It was jokingly said that to be an orthopod you had to wear a size 5 hat and a 44 jacket. Yes, there were a few jocks in the crowd but they were outnumbered by very intelligent non-jock types. Shortly after I entered orthopedics its reputation soared and it is now one of the most highly respected and well-compensated specialties in medicine. It attracts the brightest students in the class. Timing is everything!

Several days after I graduated from medical school (May, 72), Barbara gave birth to our first child, a beautiful baby girl named Melissa (from "Sweet Melissa" by The Allman Brothers). I was a "doc" and "pop" within a week. I loved holding Melissa in my arms but didn't like changing her dirty diapers of which there were many. Luckily, Pampers had just been invented.

Melissa was intellectually precocious and spoke in sentences at an early age. She was also an expert in crawling on all fours. She was so good at it that she refused to stand and walk. The doctors assured us she would eventually walk when she was ready. She finally gave up crawling and has been walking ever since.

When it came time to pick an internship I decided not to take a straight surgical internship like everybody else. I felt I was going to be doing surgery for the rest of my life so I decided to learn more about medicine while it was still possible. The mixed internship program combined both medicine and surgery. I learned to read EKG's, chest X-rays and diagnose and treat medical diseases with the best of them. As a result I had a better understanding of the patient than most other surgical residents did. While an intern in medicine, I was very highly regarded by my superiors and asked to reconsider my decision to go into orthopedics and instead become an internal medical doctor. But I never lost sight of what I really enjoyed most, which was orthopedics. However, I continued reading the New England Journal of Medicine (the bible of medical research) for many years until it became too esoteric to understand. Now, it is like reading a foreign language.

As a student and intern, I rotated through my favorite part of the hospital--the ER. There was usually nonstop action including actual gunfights in the hallways. Patients were coming in half-dead with knife wounds in the chest or their intestines hanging out and we were expected to keep them alive and patch them up as if nothing ever happened. It was notorious for being jampacked, bulging at the seams with patients and was referred to as the "zoo". For these reasons it was the most exciting area in the hospital to work. ER doctors were paid on an hourly basis nowhere near what they deserve, otherwise I would have gone into this specialty. While rotating through the department, I found it a particular challenge to try to empty out the entire ER. This was a feat that was rarely accomplished. I am proud to say that I was one of the very few doctors who were able to do it. How did I accomplish this feat? As soon as I arrived, I would write several dozen prescriptions for Darvon, the pain medicine of the moment, and Keflex, the most popular antibiotic. This way I had the scripts ready to hand out for the two most common medical problems I would see that day, severe pain and some type of infection. Also, I was able to sew up wounds faster than anybody else. I wish there were a category for this talent in the Guinness book of records. It was in the ER that my talent for surgery was confirmed. Other doctors who happened to observe my work often told me I should definitely become a surgeon. I had the ER rolling like an assembly line. The nurses had never seen this type of efficient management and did not know what to think. Some were offended by my efficiency and actually preferred the place to be like a zoo. They were upset that it was quiet and under control. I developed a reputation. On the days I did not work, the place was a jungle as usual. Although doctors are some of the smartest people, many don't have management skills or, for that matter, common sense. Their minds are too busy understanding complicated scientific problems. This is exemplified in business, where they are notorious for losing money. If they are so smart why are they the worst investors? This is a rhetorical question but my answer is that most people are talented in only one area. I like to think that I was gifted with several talents. Now on to orthopedics!

After deciding that I was going to enter orthopedics, I had to choose where to do my residency training. I applied to several programs including the Mecca of orthopedics, The Joint Disease Hospital, where I had my knee surgery ten years earlier. At Joint Disease, I would be a very, very small fish in a large pond and would have to ask permission to sneeze or cough. Instead, I decided to enter the program at Kings County Hospital where I would be a big "Charlie the Tuna" since I was already infamous from my ER stint. KCH was a great place to train for two reasons. First, every type of pathology walked through those doors. Second, you were given almost complete control of the management of the patient. This helped you learn how to think independently and develop your own way of tackling even the most difficult medical and surgical problems. Nobody was looking over your shoulder and giving you orders, unless you requested it. It was exactly the kind of place I needed since I always had difficulty taking orders and kissing up to my superiors. However, because of the lack of supervision, and lack of experience, mistakes were frequently made. I doubt that the patients were given the best medical care under these circumstances, but it is certainly a good place to learn your craft.

The residency program was only three years having just been reduced from the standard four years. I think the change was made to fill the need for more orthopedists. This meant that I cut three full years off my total education, one year in junior high (the SP), one in college (3 years) and now one in orthopedic residency. I saved another two years by not entering the armed services. When I started private practice at age 28, I was the youngest orthopedist in recent times. I was called "the boy surgeon".

As a resident, I became an obsessive-compulsive with regard to orthopedics. I wanted to learn everything there was to know and perform the most difficult surgery so that I could be the best. I read vociferously, went to every conference, and attended the many conventions. I applied all my energies to this endeavor and searched for the most difficult and unusual cases I could find. For instance, I saw a person walking in front of the hospital that had a severe bowing of both legs. I approached him, asked about his legs, and convinced him to have a consultation and X-ray. The pictures revealed one of the worst cases of rickets that anyone had ever seen. It was amazing that he was able to walk at all. I offered to straighten his legs but he was so used to his condition that he refused. Through the years I developed an excellent reputation at the hospital and was considered by my professors to be one of the best residents to complete the program.

During my last year, while I was a chief resident, I performed groundbreaking surgery, which resulted in my being asked to appear on TV. I performed the first bilateral (both right and left) ankle replacement and the first total elbow replacement in the country. Just before the elbow surgery I contacted several newspapers to make them aware of this procedure. The next day, NBC news with Frank Fields and Tom Snyder called and asked to tape the elbow replacement surgery. Of course I had to obtain consent from the patient who looked like a homeless alcoholic. He said I would have to pay him to sign. I asked him "how much" hoping he would not ask for much more than a few hundred dollars. What a complete turnaround, I was paying him to perform surgery! To my surprise he only asked for $10. To prove what a great guy I really was, I gave him $20.

The next day Channel 4 News set up the cameras in the OR and taped the operation while I gave a running commentary. The tape was aired that Sunday night on "Prime Time" and I received my fifteen minutes of fame. The newswires picked it up and the story was published in newspapers around the country and aired on the radio as well. I received numerous phone calls, most of them asking for further information, but several patients did come to me for surgery. The problem was, I did not get paid extra for these patients. As a resident I received a straight salary and that was it. What good is fame without fortune? With regard to the elbow patient, the procedure went extremely well, but the patient never returned for a follow-up. I am sure that if there were a problem, he would have definitely returned. Good luck wherever you are and I hope your new elbow is still working.

The ankle joint replacement was performed on a 30 year-old postal worker who developed necrosis (destruction) of one of the bones in the ankle. This occurred as a result of taking large doses of Prednisone (a steroid drug), which he needed to prevent kidney transplant rejection. Nobody knows why this type of complication occurs. After performing the ankle surgery I wrote a paper which was published in an orthopedic journal. The newsmedia picked up the article and published it nation wide. Without even knowing it my name was published in the World Book Encyclopedia Yearbook. Several years later an old friend contacted me and told me about the article. What a surprise! I did not believe it until she sent me a copy. Another fifteen minutes of fame sans (without) fortune!

In my last year of residency I had to decide what I was going to do after I graduate. I survived six years at Kings County Hospital, became a lean, mean, orthopedic machine, and was ready to enter the real world. Although, I've heard it is a small world, it is actually very large when you don't know where to go. I narrowed my choices down to the East Coast, West Coast, or Florida. I also had to decide whether I wanted to go into private practice or stay in academics. In addition, if I entered private practice, did I want to join a group or go solo? All these questions needed to be answered within the next few months. The opportunities were endless. In my typical, obsessive fashion I went to work and starting making thousands of phone calls and sending volumes of letters. I felt I had a phone growing out of my ear. I should have hired a secretary. Barbara could not help since she was busy as a mother, a law student and was pregnant. You could say her plate was full.

After careful consideration I decided to leave the cozy world known as academia and go into the ruthless world of private practice. I could always teach at a university on a part time basis if I needed a break from the real world. Besides, private practice was much more lucrative. I took a dozen interviews with group practices and realized I would be low man on the totem pole and would have to take orders from the other doctors in the group. I am very good at giving orders but not so good at taking them. It would have been much easier to go into an already existing practice but I would rather feel the great sense of accomplishment derived from starting up a new practice and watching it grow. This was my plan.

Now that I resolved two out of the three problems, I had to decide where in the world to open my practice. First I ruled out Florida. I was told there is a doctor on every corner and I never did like constant hot weather or living with "seasoned" citizens. They drive too slowly. From my previous experience in St. Louis, I knew I would not return to the Midwest. California was a great place to visit but it lacked the energy and culture that was available in N.Y. Besides, I never mastered the art of "channeling" and I am not fond of alfalfa sprouts. I also preferred the changing of seasons which does not exist in the land of sunshine. It gives perspective to your life. I enjoy the rebirth of nature in the spring; the rustic beauty of the fall; taking walks on the beach in the summer, and the snowy holidays of the winter. Don't get me wrong! I hate the blustery, frigid days of winter and the disgustingly hot humid days of summer. My name is not Henry David Thoreau, in case you forgot.

As it turned out it was fortunate that I did not go into practice in California, since it was one of the first states to be overtaken by the HMO's. Those are the big insurance companies that invade each state so they can force lower fees, refuse proper patient care, and drastically reduce the number of patients sent to specialists. As a result there are doctors there who are driving cabs to supplement their income. It was many years later that HMO's became prevalent in the East.

I decided to stay in the N.Y. metro area and began my search for the right opportunity. Every orthopod I spoke to complained about the fierce competition in his location and suggested that I look someplace else. Finally, I called someone in Southampton who told me I should go further East. The only place east was the Atlantic Ocean and I already knew my services were not needed there.

I continued to persevere with my search and I got the name of a town from the Suffolk County Medical Society. They did a demographic study, which found that there was a need for my specialty in a small town I had never heard of called Lindenhurst. There had previously been an orthopedist in this town several years ago but he moved to the West Coast and left a void. The medical society gave me a great idea by suggesting I call several of the general practice doctors in the area. I realized they would be more honest than other orthopods. These doctors said there was a critical need for me and they would immediately send me patients. That was all I needed to hear. The next step was to visit the town and look for suitable office space. Barbara and I went there on a sunny spring day and it was charming. It was not rich and pretentious but, middle class, clean, tree-lined streets, no slums and had a quaint Main street with mom and pop type stores. Only later did I find out it was famous for two things-the most lesbian bars and the worst hairdos. They were also in the running for the most nail salons on one street. Lindenhurst had a small doctor's row where office space happened to be available. Everything was falling into place and all signs pointed to Lindenhurst. It was "beshert" (meant to be).

The town had a large population of Italians, Irish, and Germans with a sprinkling of Jews. They were mostly working class people such as firemen, policemen, postal workers, and the like. This was the best group to have as patients since they immediately respected me as a doctor and usually followed my directions without asking a million questions. I really enjoyed the little old Italian ladies with their thick accents who had lived there for 20 years but sounded as if they had just arrived in America. They reminded me of my grandma, Bessie, who despite living in this country for 60 years, still spoke mostly Yiddish and could hardly put a sentence together in English.

I always liked the Italian language; it reminded me of opera. I even recommended that my children take Italian in school. Wendy and Josh actually did. Wendy eventually received the Italian award for the best student in the school even though she was the only student in the class that was not Italian. Josh, on the other hand managed to piss-off the teacher, but still ended up with a decent average.

I signed a three-year lease and began renovating the office. I installed new walls and wallpaper, put down floors, painted and decorated in anticipation of the big day. After many, many years of preparation I finally put up my shingle (so to speak) on July 1, 1976. Unfortunately, I was unable to participate in the celebration of the 200th anniversary of America, as I was too busy with opening my office. There were events taking place all over the city. Yes, the many sacrifices one must make.

During the first few weeks I visited a number of doctor's offices in the area, introducing myself, and I sent out a truckload of announcements. I hired a secretary and was officially open for business. Nobody showed up until a friend, who worked in the pharmacy around the corner, came in with a complaint of a sprained ankle. I don't know if he really injured his ankle or was he just doing me a favor by walking in. He complained enough and insisted that I apply a cast. He was my official first patient and the only patient for the entire day. My discouragement soon vanished since I was scheduled to be on call over the July 4th weekend, which was notorious for being extremely busy. The weather was perfect so people were outdoors drinking, partying, playing sports, and getting injured. The patients I treated in the ER would have to come to my office for follow up care. As a result I started getting busy and after several months I had a steady flow of patients. Within a year, I had a flourishing practice that continued to grow for another 20 years.

While I built up my practice, I maintained a part time academic affiliation by becoming a clinical instructor at Nassau County Hospital in their orthopedic residency-training program. I felt as a doctor, I had a duty to teach and contribute my ideas. I participated in conferences, taught surgery to the residents. and continued to write articles for the orthopedic journals. This was quite an accomplishment for a doctor to do it all; have a private practice, make contributions to the medical literature and participate in academia.

The idea for one of my papers came to me while I was a resident although I waited until now to put it in writing. I was called in the middle of the night to see an elderly lady who had fallen out of bed and dislocated her shoulder. Normally, I would wait for an X-ray and have the nurse administer Valium to relax the muscles around the shoulder in order to put it back into place. Since it was 3 AM and I wanted to get some sleep, I decided to try a new method, which was never reported. While she was still in her chair, I walked behind her, placed my forearm into her armpit, with my other hand I pulled on her arm and levered the head of the humerus (upper arm bone) back into the socket. The idea for this maneuver came to me instinctively, and out of necessity, which we all know is the "mother of invention". My technique was relatively painless and non-traumatic compared to the others that are written about in the textbook. It took all of 5 seconds to put the joint back in place. Now, I could go back to my room and get some sleep.

At first I thought I might get into trouble for not going through proper protocol. When you try something new you invariably break old rules. Innovators are rule breakers! Several months later I realized I had developed a new technique that others may want to learn and use. First, I had to figure out the biomechanical reason for its success. Then, I wrote the article, which was accepted for publication immediately. Not only was my paper published but a picture of me performing the maneuver was also included. The technique was called the Manes maneuver and I received another 15 minutes of fame. Doctors from all over the world including Russia, India and Israel requested copies of my article. Again I achieved immortality but where was the money?

PHOTO GALLERY

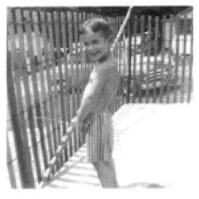

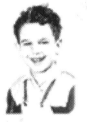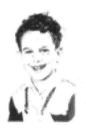

AGE 6-WHAT ME WORRY?

11952-AGE 4-Nature Calls

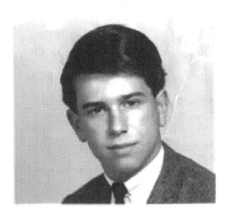

16-High School Graduation

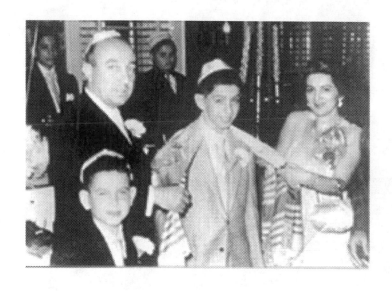

1956 -Age 8- Brother Ted's Bar Mitzvah-one big happy family

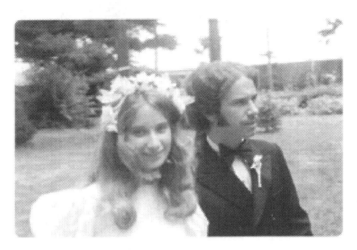

1970-age 22-My Wedding Day-Aug 30

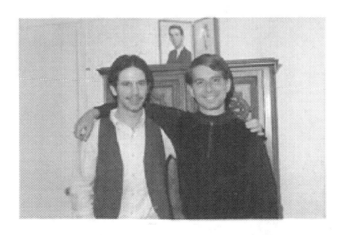

1974- Ted and me. Don't we look like Twins?

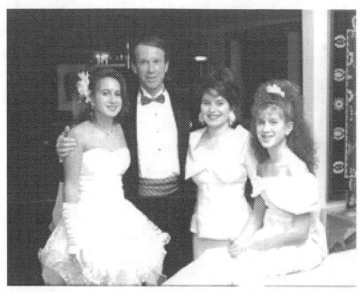

1989-Wendy's Bar Mitzvah. I could stay in this year forever

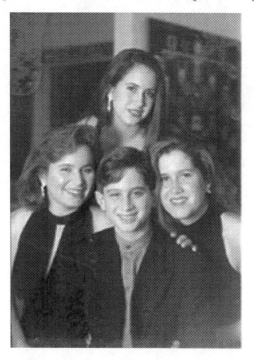

Josh's Bar Mitzvah- They are getting older and so am I

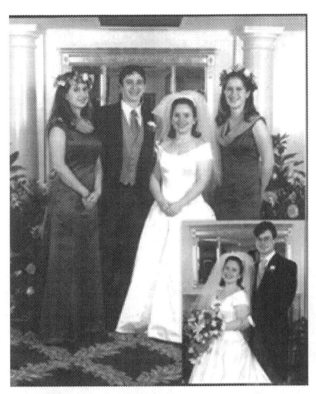

1998-Melissa & Michaels Wedding in London

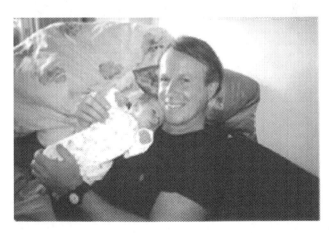

2001-Grandpa Harvey and Jacob

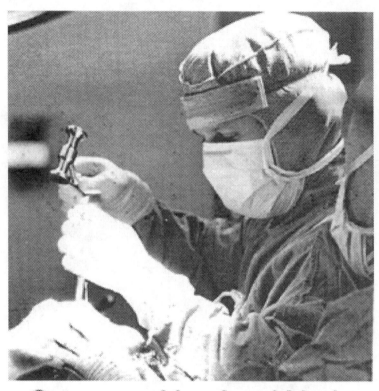

Surgeon Hard at Work

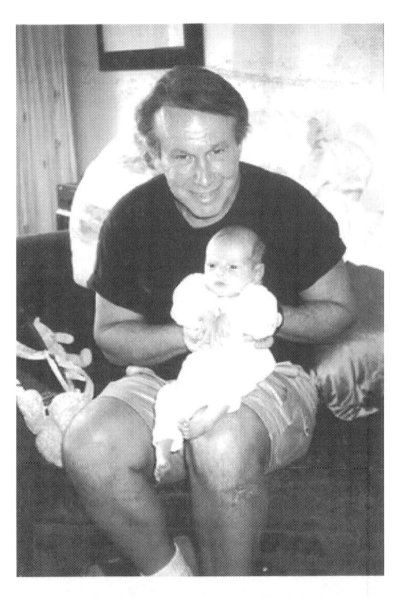

The Present & Future
Grandpa & Grandson

CHAPTER 4: THE DOCTOR & FAMILY MAN

However, along with my newfound success, I experienced tragedy. Barbara was pregnant with our second child during my residency and was about to give birth. She had already gone through one delivery with no problem and was ready for another easy-as-pie birth. I took a video camera to the birthing room, which in those days was unheard of. I was going to show the world how Barbara made giving birth look so easy. No video was ever taken though. She had gone into labor so we rushed to the hospital. The resident doctor had trouble hearing the heart beat but assured us that everything was O.K. Our private obstetrician arrived 45 minutes later and again did not hear the heartbeat. Immediately, action was taken to deliver the baby. He did not want to do a C-section so as not to mark up Barbara's body. They did a vaginal delivery and the baby, Jonah, was delivered stillborn. The next day we walked out of the hospital not with a bouncing baby, but with a heavy heart and empty handed. We buried the baby, just the two of us, in a cemetery, even though we were told it was not necessary. Why did God do this to us? I know I committed many sins, but I thought I was basically a good person, and Barbara was a saint. Although I would like to believe there is a God, when bad things happen to good people, belief becomes much more difficult.

Obviously there is no good explanation for this tragedy. It caused us to retreat from the world. In his memory Barbara created some of her best paintings, "Jonah and the Whale", and "The Carousel". The only uplifting aspect that may have come out of this tragedy was that in some way it inspired Barbara to have not one but several more children in the future. Secondly, it made her reevaluate her life goals and inspired her to take on a new challenge by returning to school and pursue a career in law. Jonah will always be remembered in our hearts. I believe part of his soul inhabits our other children.

It took a couple of long and depressing years before Barbara could conceive another child. Her fertility level bottomed out, probably as a result of what had happened. After trying unsuccessfully for one year, we decided to go to a fertility expert who did numerous tests on both of us. The sperm count test was the most fun, masturbating in a cup. And yes they do have magazines for your perusal. My count was on the upper end of curve. What a macho man! Apparently, Barbara's tubes were slightly blocked so the doctor blew them out with an air gun. She was also given the fertility pill, Clomid. With a lot of effort on my part, she was pregnant the following month, with our darling angel, Wendy.

Wendy was the most desired child on the planet. She was beautiful and continues to be a source of joy. However, when she was born her nose was bent to óne side marring her otherwise perfect face. While I fed her a bottle (in between Barbara's breast feedings) and held her in my arms I would apply gentle pressure on her nose in the opposite direction. Eventually her nose straightened out and she now has one of the most perfect proboscises, in America. I am not sure if my intervention was the key but I like to think I helped Mother Nature. By the way, Wendy was not named after the hamburger chain, but from a combination of several other Wendy's. There was Wendy the "wench", a Harpur college cutie who had long straight hair down to her waist and wore high leather boots. Next was Peter Pan's Wendy. Let's not forget Wendy the good witch in Little Lulu comic books. And last was a childhood friend of Barbara's who had the same birthday. Wendy will not admit it but I think she does like the name.

Several months later, without even trying, Barbara was pregnant with Natasha. She was the second most wanted child on this planet. She was born with a smile on her face that is still there till this day. She was such a beautiful child that she was asked to model on several occasions. She is the only child to follow in my footsteps to become a doctor. Although the field of medicine has changed dramatically in the past decade, it is still a very rewarding and prestigious career to enter.

At this point, I am the father of three girls, no boys. They are all fantastic, but what is a man without having a son? One night, several years after Natasha was born, Barbara insisted that we conjugate. This command was out of character for her. She never was the initiator. That night she had an intuition that she would become pregnant with a male child. She practically guaranteed it! I was extremely skeptical and did not believe her for a minute, but what would I lose by trying? After all, making babies is not hard work. I did not forget that night and waited in anticipation to see if her intuition was correct. Would you believe two weeks later she missed her period and announced she was very pregnant. Still, I was convinced the baby was going to be another female and was preparing myself for 4 girls. That would be even more difficult to live down than three. I probably would not even send out an announcement. An orthopedic friend of mine also had four girls. I started to believe that orthopods, as macho as they are, were only capable of siring girls; but I wanted to be proven wrong.

A sonogram was performed at three months and there it was--a penis! Now I know what it felt like to be on cloud ten (nine was already occupied by Barbara). The test is not 100% accurate but pretty close. When Josh was born and the findings were confirmed, I felt my life was complete and God was good again. After the stillborn, all I really cared about was having a normal, healthy child, but having a boy was the icing on the cake. He was named inadvertently after my living father, Sidney (Hebrew name, Joshua) and purposely given the Hebrew name of Barbara's deceased father, Murray. We liked the name Joshua, because it was both biblical and cool. In slang it means, "to fool", as in joshing around. Only later did we realize how popular the name had become.

I must say something more about my children or I will be banished to the doghouse forever. First of all, they give my life meaning and purpose more than anything else does. My life would be very empty without them. By not having children I believe a person does not complete the cycle of life. Although they require a great deal of work, they provide enormous pleasure in return. Each of my children is very different. In describing them I must be very diplomatic. If I don't give equal time to each, it will just provide them with ammunition for the psychotherapist. When we share private time together I make each one think that I love them the best. When we are in a group, I show no such favoritism. They will never know which one I prefer. Actually, I don't see how a parent can love one child over another. Each one brings something different to the table.

Melissa is the oldest and wisest. She was mature beyond her years and was able to engage in adult conversation by the time she was 5 years old. Her intellectual curiosity was enormous. She asked millions of questions about everything around her including "why is the sky blue, daddy"? I was well prepared for questions asked by the other children, thanks to her. She was extremely organized, made long lists of things to do and was disappointed if she was unable to finish what was on the list. Her intelligence and maturity was confirmed when she entered kindergarten where she was way ahead of the other children. We spoke to the principal about having her skip a grade. His reluctance was predictable but after an in depth interview he agreed and said that she was the only student he ever permitted to skip. Another especially proud moment was when she received her SAT scores, which were the highest in her high school. It gave me bragging rights for the next six months. Aside from her intellect she was also very charming and beautiful and frequently had boyfriends knocking down her door. She left a long line of broken hearts.

One of her biggest achievements was being accepted to pursue a degree at Oxford University, one of only a few students chosen from the U.S. I never dreamed a child of mine would receive such an honor. Since she was too young to attend right after high school and was interested in diplomacy, she applied and was accepted to the Foreign Services Department at Georgetown University. For diplomacy, this school was the best in the country. While she was there she became friendly with numerous foreign diplomats especially from Eastern Europe. She was able to get all of them to participate in a roundtable discussion about the future of Eastern Europe, of which she was the chairperson. I don't how she did it but I do not think even the U.N. could have accomplished such a feat at that time.

However she did one thing that really upset me. Upon leaving for England she promised she would come home to the U.S. right after graduation. This never happened. As predicted she met her future husband, Michael Collett, another student at Oxford, and took up residence in London. Michael is a handsome, very intelligent, tall and lithe chap with fine facial features. Upon our first meeting he had the gentleman reserve and polish of a typical Englishman, which was in contrast to Melissa, who was charming but had the forwardness of a typical New Yorker. As a couple they exhibited a good example of the laws of magnetism (opposites attract). To their mutual benefit, over the years, Michael has become more aggressive while Melissa has become more reserved. They have been together for more than five years and tied the proverbial "knot" two years ago with a wedding that was right out of a fairy tale only instead of driving up in a horse drawn carriage, they substituted it with a white "Rolls Royce". She works as a solicitor while he is a barrister. Translation-they are both attorneys! She frequently calls, and travels to N.Y. several times a year, but I still wish she were closer to home. However, it does give me an excuse to travel to London on a regular basis.

My next child, Wendy is beautiful, smart and was a godsend. However, at one year of age when most babies have around six teeth in their mouth she still did not have any. Not one! I brought her to the dentist who agreed there were no teeth; she was all gums. Before anyone panicked the dentist decided to take an X-ray. She had plenty of teeth, but they were still hiding within her gums. She did not need to be fitted with false teeth. What a relief!

Wendy was also the most sensitive and edgy sibling in the family. Most of the time she is friendly and upbeat but occasionally I recommend keeping your distance. It must be genetic because her father is the same way. To her credit she has many accomplishments. She participated in Karate and was one of the best in the class. She drew the best election posters the high school had ever seen. She excelled in piano. She even excelled in the French horn. She never told anybody about all the after school activities she was involved in. At graduation from the 6th grade she was called up to the stage for each of these activities. Her name was mentioned more than any other student in her class. It was. Wendy, Wendy, Wendy, at least 8 times! She had a little pixie smile on her face each time she was called. I was surprised and extremely proud.

At high school graduation her name was mentioned as one of the top 20 students in her class and was the winner of the award for the best student in Italian. I was especially proud of her when she was accepted to one of the best colleges in the country, Cornell. I always wanted to go there but my grades were not high enough. Wendy went there in my place. When it comes to boys, she has it all, brains and beauty but is very selective. She has dated more than both her sisters put together but is still looking for her perfect match.

Wendy recently came to a crossroads in her life. In college, she majored in restaurant management and after graduation landed a very sought after job with a prestigious firm. Unfortunately she had to work long hours and weekends without adequate compensation. She finally had enough and decided to quit. At this point she had to choose a new career path and decide where to go to school. This was a pivotal point in her life. The stress was so great that she developed a hyperactive thyroid condition. After thorough consideration of all her choices she finally decided to pursue a Masters degree in education at the George Washington University in D.C. She believed that being a teacher is a very important job where she would be able to help young students as well as use her intelligence and communication skills. Besides the teacher shortage was getting worse while salaries were going up. Congratulations on a smart choice.

Natasha is my favorite third child. She is also beautiful, smart, popular, and funny. Amazingly, nothing seems to bother her. When faced with a disappointment, which was rare, she would quickly put it in the past and moved on. School was a breeze; she hardly studied and was still in the top 20 students in her class. Combined with her academic skills, she was also well liked by her peers and teachers. She excelled in all subjects and was recommended to do research for the Westinghouse Scholarship, a coveted award. She also won the Social Studies award at graduation from high school.

Tasha will never let me live down a dirty trick I played on her when she was around 8. We were walking on the boardwalk in Coney Island and looking over the railing down to the beach, which was only about six feet below. Since she was quite the daredevil I dared her to hang from my hands over the railing of the boardwalk. Of course she took my dare and while she was hanging in the air about 2 feet above the sand I let her go. I knew she would be surprised, fall to the sand below, and not hurt herself. But since she was not expecting it, she let out a loud scream. When she hit the sand she started crying as if in pain but I knew she didn't really hurt herself. She learned an important lesson that day--not to trust anybody, especially her father.

When she was 12, she went to acting and dancing camp. On visiting day, the entire camp put on a show for the parents. They picked Tasha to perform a leading tap-dance number that was the highlight of the show. She did such a terrific job that she ended up winning the award for the best dancer. She was also an excellent ballet dancer (living up to her name) but decided not to pursue a career in that area.

Tasha graduated University of Pennsylvania with honors and is now in medical school at The University of Buffalo. She will carry on the legacy of medicine in the Manes family started by yours truly. She is finishing her second year, which is still mostly academic. In the third year she will participate in direct patient care and put everything she learned in the past two years to the test. She is still not sure what area in medicine to specialize, but I don't think it will be orthopedics. She is currently going out with another med-student named Alex for the past year. He is a friendly, handsome, very bright boy with a terrific future.

Josh is my pride and joy and my favorite son. As the youngest and the only male, he was in an enviable position being catered to by everyone else around. I was not sure how smart he was until he was about 5 years old when Billy Joel's famous song "We Didn't Start the Fire" became popular. The song was a complex monologue about recent historical events and personalities stated in a somewhat staccato manner. There were many names, events and places mentioned in the song that were completely unknown to Josh at the time. One day he began singing the words to the entire song. I was astonished! He must have had a photographic memory. From that time on I knew he was very bright. He was so bright that sometimes I called him "Sunny".

Several years later he was given an I.Q. test, which revealed he was truly intellectually gifted. I had four intellectually gifted and talented children. I guess the milkman had very good genes. I am a Jew with the luck of the Irish. Josh's parents and siblings were a hard act to follow for anyone but he rose to the occasion. He was the only one in the family to really excel in music. He played the drums so well he was selected to the "All County" band. He was the leader of the band in the play "Grease" and was singled out by name and complimented by the music teacher. He also taught himself to play the guitar and the bass well enough to play either of them in a band.

He is also a terrific athlete having won the top fitness award at his school for five years in a row. He is a pro on roller-blades and skis. Jumping over barrels and going down long flights of stairs backwards are a few examples of his talent on "blades". On skis he is able to conquer double black diamonds with the best of them. Last but certainly not least, after many years of training he became one of the youngest black belts in Karate in the country.

In spite of all his talents, when Josh entered high school he had a problem. He was one of the shortest kids in the class. All his friends were a head taller. I would measure his height almost on a daily basis and chart it on a graph. He was growing very slowly. I decided to perform a bone age analysis, which indicated that he was delayed in growth by at least one year. That meant his normal growth spurt was going to occur later than his peers. I tried to allay his fears but was still very concerned that everybody around him was taller. It took awhile but eventually he started to sprout up and is now over 5'10". No stretching machines were necessary.

Josh, started to take an interest in architecture and design at an early age. I was also interested in this area but did not have the talent to pursue it. To find out if he indeed had talent, he decided to study architecture during his high school summer vacation at a special program for students at The University of Miami. Once again, he excelled, so he decided to enter a college program, which specializes in architecture, at the highly respected Washington University in St. Louis.

Now that I have finished writing about my children I am emotionally drained and have to take a break. Be back soon! Thank you for your patience.

I'm back! As a family, we did everything together. Movies, museums, vacations, restaurants, everything! I wanted my children to be exposed to and experience as much as possible. They will never complain to me, "daddy, how come we never did this or that"? I did not want them to lead sheltered lives like most suburban kids. They had culture up the whazzoo. We would frequently go to the more interesting areas of the city like Soho and The Village, where people watching was the main event. Ski trips in the Catskills was also on the agenda every winter. The only time we did not do things as a family was when the kids went to camp in the summer. Everybody needs a break!

While the children were still toddlers, I decided that we should have a place for weekend getaways, so I bought a really cute house in a community called Oak Beach. It was a two bedroom wooden house that was on the water and had its own private beach. We were able to go out on the bay, fishing, boating, and swimming or when the tide was low, we could actually walk to the middle of the bay on a sand bar. Coming from the tenements of Brooklyn, this was quite a lifestyle change for me. The house was very quaint but always needed fixing. While the kids were having fun I was working my little butt off painting and repairing. But it was fun to sleep in a different bed and wake up to the sounds of the ocean. There was only one place to go for breakfast in the morning. It was an old, dinky restaurant and falling apart, but had the best pancakes in the world.

From the beach house we frequently went to Robert Moses beach which was only five minutes away. We loved to walk along the shore to Fire Island, about 45 minutes away. Because the kids were so small, especially Josh, it seemed like the walk lasted forever. I helped each of them by carrying them on my shoulders part of the way. It was beautiful, invigorating, and good exercise. For part of the walk it was necessary to pass by one of the few nude beaches in the country. At first the nudies were few and stayed all the way in the back. Ten years later the same beach was filled with thousands of them right up front and in your face. I would not have minded except that most of the bodies were quite ugly and out of shape. My kids didn't seem to mind and would giggle most of the way. I tried to convince myself that this was an educational experience for them and not obscene. I hope I was right!

When the children got older they did not want to go to the beach house anymore. They preferred to play with their friends and not hang out with their parents. I don't blame them, parents are so boring! The house stayed in the family for 15 years but it was time to sell. It was a sad day in the history of the Manes family when I sold the house. Fortunately, I quadrupled my money.

One hot summer day when we were on our way back from the beach house we decided to stop at a new clam bar restaurant that had just opened. We walked in (the place was completely empty) and sat down. The manager immediately came over and told us that we were not allowed to stay because I was wearing a tank top shirt, which was prohibited. My wife was also wearing a tank top but the rule only applied to men. He said there was a sign posted in the front of the restaurant "no tank tops" and he was not going to serve us. I asked him to please make an exception since there was nobody else there and we were very hungry. In a loud and mean tone of voice he said "no". I was extremely annoyed that he was being so stubborn and denying food to my children. In anger, on the way out I ripped the sign off the wall. All of us ran to the parking lot and into the safety of our car and tried to make a quick getaway. The manager and the employees came out after us and tried to stop my car, unsuccessfully. I almost ran them over. The kids were rattled and on one hand I was embarrassed about my actions but on the other I felt justified. My family berated me for creating a scene.

The following week while I was relaxing at home and the incident was long forgotten a police officer knocked on my door. He said the manager filed a complaint against me and I owed $150 for the broken sign. I was ready to explode but I replied in a calm manner (after counting to 10) that if he insisted on collecting for the sign I would bring a sex discrimination lawsuit against him so fast that it would make his head spin. This was in the early 1980's when these suits were made popular by women libbers. The officer listened and fortunately left without a reply. He must have been a friend of the manager and was just trying to intimidate me. I never heard about the matter again except when my kids bring it up to embarrass me. Their daddy is a rebel and will never change.

CHAPTER 5: SHIT HAPPENS

At this point, I am 35, have 4 children, a successful career, live in a big house, drive a luxury car, and have a bright looking future. It was a long and arduous struggle but the hard work and perseverance paid off big time. From the mean-streets of Brooklyn which seemed like a lifetime ago to multi-millionaire. I was more successful than in my wildest dreams. Sadly, just as I was peaking, my life began to unravel. Not on purpose and not because I had a subconscious wish to fail. As far as I can tell it was a result of a few bad decisions combined with a lot of bad luck. Being surrounded by jealous, insecure people, who were out to castrate me, didn't help. Hey, I am not going to take all the blame! A dark cloud made an appearance over my head, affecting both my marriage and career. The only consolation was that I was in good company. Many successful people go through a similar experience. Even the Bible states, "God giveth and taketh away". You just have to look at our recent presidents-Johnson, Nixon, Carter, Ford, Bush, and Clinton. Each one, after having reached the top was taken down, some worse than others were. The news is filled with successful people whose fortunes have changed.

It started when I began to question the goals in my life and what direction I should take. "Mid-life crisis" was knocking at my door and trying to break it down. The crisis was not just in my mind but was aided and abetted by external events. First, my wife decided to put her libido on hold. When I complained, her answer was that I should go elsewhere for such pleasures. So I did! Once I was bitten by the cheating-bug, it was impossible to turn back. From that moment, we both knew our marriage would never be the same. I did not want to leave my children while they were young so despite my dissatisfaction, I stayed in the marriage for many more years and tried a number of times to resolve the differences that we had but to no avail. Counseling was attempted but unsuccessful. There were other problems in the marriage that I will discuss later.

I thought if I tried something new, I would not focus on my declining marriage. I had just returned from a Club Med vacation where inhibitions are thrown to the wind and decided to pursue a career in acting. I believed my movie star looks (ha, ha) and charismatic personality would make me an instant star. I signed up for acting lessons at a local theater where they are good at teaching you to act like a tree or a zoo animal, among other things. Actually, you have to dig down into yourself to really act out a part. In order to display sadness, depression, elation, or surprise, you are supposed to conjure up memories of these feeling from past experiences. It's akin to therapy. Many actors continue to feel the emotions for some time after playing their roles. At the end of the semester each student performs a part in a play that has been selected by the instructor. I played the mean boss of Willie Loman in "Death of a Salesman", and a comedic role in "Plaza Suite", by Neil Simon.

After taking lessons for a year I tried to land a real part in a full length production and ended up at the Commack Y playing a few minor roles in the play "Funny Girl". I had to do a little singing, a little dancing, and a little acting (very little). Next, I was picked to play the lead role in a murder mystery, "Catch Me if You Can". I was the murderer so it wasn't much of a stretch for me. Everybody who saw the play said I did a terrific job (such liars). I thought I was on the way to fame and fortune until I tried to get a part that paid money. What good is fame without fortune? I auditioned for many roles and kept on getting rejected. Occasionally I would get a "call-back" and my confidence would surge. Still, I never landed anything more than being in the chorus, which was not for me. I decided to end my acting career shortly thereafter. I rationalized that the fact that they never appreciated me was not because of lack of talent, but my lack of showbiz connections. I needed to find some excuse.

At the same time that my marriage was on the rocks, I began having professional problems. As a pushy New Yorker, I had difficulty with authority and bureaucrats who blindly follow stupid rules and try to enforce them no matter how ridiculous. I especially become annoyed when the rules get in my way. How dare they! Although I have been told that I could charm the birds out of the trees, I frequently come off as arrogant and unfriendly. The truth is I don't have patience. I think and move quickly and efficiently and become impatient with slow thinking and slow moving people. Unfortunately, they are in the majority. I learned early on not to take "no" for an answer. That philosophy helped me to reach the top but I also made many enemies en route. In particular, the nurses and administrators are always the enemy. I have been reported for breaking the rules more times than there are grains of sand at the beach. I agree with Woody Allen that some people are above the law and have the right to make their own rules. He certainly lived up to his own words by ignoring the taboo of incest and marrying his own daughter. Personally I don't think I would go that far but his idea does have some merit.

The first big screw-up occurred in the ER when I was just about to repair a bad finger laceration. The nurse said I could not proceed because they were expecting a major trauma patient and they needed all the nurses available for him. I said to myself, this is ridiculous because chances are the patient was not in such a dire emergency and I didn't need any nurses to help me anyway. I started the case and told her that if I was in anybody's way she could stop me. I continued to work and at about the time I finished the patient arrived. Perfect timing, I thought. Everything was cool until the following week when I received a nasty letter from administration telling me that my privileges were suspended and I had to attend a hearing. I was devastated, but learned two valuable lessons. You better listen to the nurses because they will stab you in the back at any given notice, and that the administration was more interested in appeasing the nurses than standing up for the doctors. Unfortunately, I learned this lesson the hard way many more times. I would never accept the fact that the nurse had more power than the doctor did. After all, we were the ones who went to medical school so shouldn't we be the ones in charge? That would make sense but that was not the case.

My next infraction occurred the following year again in the ER. I was called to treat a patient with a dislocated shoulder. I put the joint back in place with no problem and ordered the post reduction X-ray. Since it would take about an hour for the films to be completed, it was standard for most ER doctors to look at these films so the treating doctor could leave. I asked the ER doctor to review the films for me. At the time he had his hands around a nurse's waist and appeared to be flirting. To my surprise he turned towards me and said "no", even though I told him that I had to go to another ER right away. His lack of cooperation was clearly evident. I reacted swiftly and called him an "asshole". Apparently, I just committed an unpardonable sin by using the "A" word. Once again I was suspended from the hospital, only this time it was permanent. It meant an immediate loss of 1/3 of my practice. In order to avoid being reported to the State, they allowed me to resign. I was young and naïve and afraid of the State so I acquiesced. Little did I know, I could have hired a lawyer, fought the suspension and probably won.

This time the silver lining theory came true I was asked to apply to another small hospital in the area that really needed an orthopedist. Not only did I quickly get on staff, but was well liked, and took over most of the orthopedic work at the hospital. I was appointed the Chief of the department shortly thereafter. This was the one hospital where my abilities were recognized and appreciated. Unfortunately, after a long run the hospital eventually closed.

Next, I got hit with what every doctor fears the most, a malpractice suit. I heard a lot about it but after being in practice for five years with a clean record, I never thought it would happen to me, until one day when I was called to treat a deep finger laceration that involved bone and tendon. It was a complicated case. While I repaired the finger there was a crowd of students around me to whom I gave a running commentary and I thought I did an excellent job of repair. The patient did not return to my office the next day as instructed but instead showed up a week later. After I removed the bandage, I noted that the finger became infected. I put the patient on antibiotics and instructed him to clean the wound and change the bandage several times a day. Again, he never returned. Apparently he went to another doctor who instead of allowing the infection to heal, decided to amputate. His decision was based on the faulty reading of the X-ray indicating bone infection instead of bone loss. Several months later I received a summons for malpractice. Had the patient returned to my office as requested or had the other surgeon properly interpreted the X-rays, the amputation and lawsuit could have been avoided. In orthopedics whenever there is a complication such as infection, or if a fracture does not properly heal, a lawsuit is frequently filed, even though it is not the fault of the surgeon. Unfortunately, the case is usually settled and the patient walks away with a windfall, while the surgeon is penalized. That is the system! I didn't create it. It sucks and should be changed but too many lawyers are getting rich as a result and they make the laws.

Through the years I developed one of the busiest practices on Long Island and took on many difficult cases. Combine that with the fact that Long Island is the most litigious area in the country and orthopedics is the most frequently sued specialty and you have the formula for a large number of malpractice suits. Eventually my insurance premium went up to over $300,000 per year. Yikes! Although they were usually unjustified, each suit chips away at your confidence and self-esteem. There have been a number of physician suicides as a result of malpractice. You must keep your perspective and focus on the good you are doing but the system makes you very cynical. On the average I treat one thousand patients per year and get sued once per year. That means I successfully treat 99.9% of my patients.

As I have said, within a short period of time, I was forced to resign from my main hospital, I experienced my first malpractice case, and my marriage was falling apart. I guess you can say my life was becoming more complex. Barbara and I were having more frequent fights. Not so much yelling, but disagreements. I was annoyed that after the children went to bed and it was time for us to communicate, she frequently would fall asleep. I complained about that many times but she didn't change. I really couldn't blame her for being tired since she worked full time as an attorney, and then came home to attend to our four kids and the house. That would make anybody tired. But I also worked hard and helped in the house. At 9 PM, I was ready to spend quality time with my spouse and was not ready to call it a day. I started getting bored and needed further stimulation. I was married for over ten years and had lived through the seven-year itch, the eight-year bitch, the nine-year witch, and the ten-year switch. We both were ready for a change, something new, and exciting. It was time to find out what else was out there. Maybe we were missing something. We decided to establish a new type of relationship where I would spend one night a week, Friday, out of the house and return the following morning. We would go our separate ways and have a private life for that one night. It was similar to taking a separate mini-vacation. For awhile the one night separation worked. The next morning we would be happy to see each other. After several years of Friday night follies, I suggested to Barbara that we stop and try to get our marriage back on track. To my great disappointment she said she enjoyed her freedom and preferred this arrangement. This was not a good sign.

I like to think that my children were not affected by this arrangement since they were usually busy anyway and I came back the next morning before they were awake. Even though the marriage was faltering, the kids were doing well and to me that was the most important thing. I wanted my children to feel they lived in a stable, loving and supportive family environment.

I was just about to celebrate my 40th birthday when I received an emergency call from my 44-year-old brother Ted. "Harvey, the doctor told me I may have leukemia". I tried to find a place to sit and digest the horrible news my brother was relating to me on the phone. As a doctor, my gut reaction was that he was overreacting to what was probably a lab error. As he further elaborated, I was thinking to myself, what if they were right. He had been feeling vague weakness in his body for several months and occasional finger numbness in both hands, but he ignored these feelings because he had just gotten a clean bill of health after a complete physical exam three months ago. A few days before the phone call he noticed a funny looking red rash on his belly and chest and finally decided to go to his doctor. The GP said he had never seen a rash quite like this and sent him to a dermatologist for lab tests. The next day, while at work, Ted got a call that his white blood count was extremely high. "Ted, don't get excited," I said. "It's probably some kind of mistake. I am going to send you to the best hematologist and I am sure he'll tell you it was a mistake".

Now I was the one getting anxious. What if it is true? He is only 44, has two young kids, is recently out of an unhappy marriage, and is starting to enjoy life as a single man. If it is true he may only have a few months to live. The next day at the hospital, after numerous tests, including a bone marrow tap, I find out the bad news. He indeed has a very aggressive form of leukemia. The good news is that he can be treated and there is a 60% chance of recovery.

A hematologist friend suggests that my brother is transferred to Sloan-Kettering, the Mecca for cancer treatment, and I immediately make all the arrangements. For the first few days after he was admitted, a party atmosphere prevailed in his room, with balloons and get well cards decorating the walls, while relatives and friends were coming and going. Even though he was subjected to different tests and had started on chemotherapy he was still feeling and looking well. In the middle of the night the next day, I got a call from the house doctor. He said that Ted couldn't breathe because he was bleeding into his lungs and needed to be intubated and put on a respirator. The bottom was beginning to fall out. Why did he suddenly start bleeding? I tried to grasp the reason for this rapid turn of events. The doctors were hedging when confronted by my questions.

I went to the hospital the next morning and he was in intensive care, unresponsive, with numerous tubes going in and out of his veins, lungs, mouth, nose, and pelvis. Now the doctors were saying he could die at any time. I was completely baffled. Everything happened so fast that he had no time to say goodbye or get his affairs in order. It was all too sudden. Two weeks later he was still in a coma, developed a serious infection, was in kidney failure, and may have had bleeding into his brain. I talked to him every day and encouraged him to stay strong and fight the disease. I whispered to him that he had lots of great things to look forward to. I was told that he could hear me in some remote area of his brain.

As my confidence in the miracles of medicine was being rapidly undermined, I added prayer to my armamentarium and believed he now was in the hands of God. Tragically, Ted died several days later.

Through this ordeal I came to recognize the irony of my powerlessness as a doctor to help my own brother in his battle against a terrible disease and saw firsthand the limitations of medicine. I think about Ted and miss him every day of my life.

My practice was still going strong in spite of all its problems and I had enough work for two other doctors. A few of my colleagues recommended that I take on another doctor in my practice. I had been on call 24/7 for the past 15 years and literally tied to my beeper. Although it would cost me $200,000 it would be well worth it to be able to have time off. Besides, by taking more ER call he may bring in some patients and pay his way. At this point I was taking ER calls at six hospitals.

I spread the word, advertised and received many replies. One of the candidates was a woman who was 6 feet tall and skinny. I could picture us walking down the hospital corridors looking like Mutt and Jeff. I am not sure why she even bothered with an interview since she was more interested in academic medicine than private practice. I also interviewed an older man, who wanted to leave the West Coast. However, I could not see hiring someone older than me to be my junior partner. I ended up with someone who had been working in a large medical clinic for several years. At first it was terrific, especially since I could turn off my beeper. Unfortunately, the luxury of a partner did not last very long, one year to be exact. He made so many mistakes that I was forced to constantly look over his shoulder. This translated into double the work for me. For example, he left a 9-inch guide pin in the pelvis of a patient that was having surgery for a fractured hip. The guide pin is supposed to be removed before closing the wound. There was no way short of major surgery to remove this pin. It was so unusual that the textbooks don't even mention this complication. Fortunately for him, but not for the patient, she died from medical complications totally unrelated to the hip. To put it mildly, he was incompetent. And yet, he quit before I could fire him and stole $40,000 worth of checks. Lawsuits went flying back and forth and eventually I received my money back. As a result of this experience I decided partnership was not for me. Instead, I would contract my practice, drop out of several hospitals, and take less ER call. When I needed coverage I hired a friend of mine, Dr. Pierre Rafiy, who was happy to oblige.

My marriage continued to unravel by the frequent arguments over unresolved issues, but my children were older and I believe in a better position to weather any storm between their parents. Melissa was a student at Oxford, Wendy started college at Cornell; and Natasha was a senior in high school with a very busy social life. My main concern was Josh who was ten years old, still a vulnerable age and likely to be affected by his parents' discord. Barbara asked me to leave. This time I didn't put up a fight although in retrospect, I should have. I told her it would be less traumatic if I left during the summer while Josh was in camp. She agreed to wait until then.

My father left the house when I was ten years old and on looking back it was probably a good thing. I believe that the independence it afforded me as a child was a maturing experience. According to Freud there is a natural tendency for a son to be in competition with his father for the mother's attention, ala Oedipus. Since Josh was surrounded by women and was the youngest, he was catered to and remained somewhat immature. By my leaving, he would become "the man" of the house. This responsibility would help him grow up. However, when he came home from camp and was informed about our separation, he developed a nervous twitch with his head. When he saw that I moved only five minutes away, was still friendly with his mother, and frequently ate dinners at the house, the twitch quickly disappeared. I believe my theory was right in that he did become more responsible and mature with time.

Initially when I move out, I lived in a small apartment above my office. It was very convenient since I could literally get out of bed and walk into my office. But that was the only benefit. The apartment itself was totally unsuit-ible for a sophisticated "man about town". What would a date think if I rought her back to this makeshift apartment? First her eyeballs would roll p into her head and then she would be out of there faster than roadrunner on eed. I had to find something better or my social life would be non-existent. quickly found the perfect apartment only five minutes from my former idence. It was modern with vaulted ceilings, lots of wall space for my art lection and had a fabulous view of a pond with geese, surrounded by ping willow trees. As soon as I walked in I knew this was the place. Did ntion it was furnished?

CHAPTER 6: MORE OF THE SAME

Until I began to slow my practice down and stop taking ER calls, I continued to pile up the malpractice cases. The vast majority arose as a result of unavoidable complications. In total, I only had 2 or 3 suits that may have resulted from my negligence. I am human and no matter how hard I try I make mistakes like everybody else. After 20 years of practice my malpractice insurance was in the highest category. At this point I decided maybe I should leave N.Y. and start over in another part of the country. I considered California and Florida. After visiting these areas and speaking to other orthopods I realized N.Y. was not so bad after all. In California, the HMOs had already made big inroads and reduced doctors' fees across the board to below one half of the usual. Also, because of the pressures from the HMOs, the specialists were seeing far fewer patients. I was told it was so bad that some doctors were actually unemployed. On the other hand Florida had such a glut of doctors, they were falling over themselves. Also, since most of the population were elderly and on Medicare, the fees were government controlled and very low. No matter how rich a patient was, and many of them are, they were not allowed to pay the doctor. So even though I was paying through the nose for insurance, I was still making a decent living especially compared to doctors in other parts of the country. I decided to stay put, and learn to sing "I Love New York". I continued to appreciate the variety of activities only available in this city. The museums, galleries, restaurants, theatre, and people are the most interesting in the world. As a single person it was also the best place to live.

Since I would stay in N.Y. I decided that maybe I should pursue another line of work and give up orthopedics. The two areas that I had a particular expertise in were the art market and the stock market. I am frequently asked how did I become interested in art considering the fact that I grew up relatively poor in a tenement in Brooklyn. My first exposure to art when I was a child were the two copies of famous paintings on the walls of my apartment, "The Blue Boy" by Gainsborough and "The Creation of Man" by Michelangelo. I would climb on a chair and study the fine details of each painting. It was fascinating to me. Even though my first love was sports, I would jump at the chance when asked to go to the Brooklyn Museum with my dad. This reaction was in contrast to my friends who were totally turned off by museums. I could never understand their lack of interest.

My interest in art continued into college where I decided to take a class in art history. After one class I was hooked. I felt a part of me was reborn. I understand what Nieztche meant when he said, "Art is the great stimulant of life". I couldn't get enough of it and signed up for more courses every semester. It was the only course I looked forward to especially after attending classes in physics, calculus, and chemistry. For each art course I was required to write a paper. The subject of my first paper was to compare two artists that I had never heard of-- Fragonard and Grueze. I located their paintings at the Met and the Frick and described their different techniques with regard to color, design, and subject matter. This was one of the rare times that I actually enjoyed writing, and it must have shown since I received an "A".

The art class was given in a large lecture hall with dozens of students. On the first day the professor asked the class if anyone was aware of an historic event that had just occurred in the art world. I knew the answer but waited to see if anyone else raised his or her hand. I was amazed that nobody knew the answer except me. I proceeded to raise my hand and told the class that a painting by Rembrandt entitled "Aristotle Contemplating the Bust of

Homer" was sold for $2.4 million. The teacher was very impressed and from that time on I knew I was destined for stardom in art history.

While studying art history I felt my creative juices flowing so I took up sculpting. I bought some clay and began working on my first piece. It was the bust of a man. I thoroughly enjoyed sculpting with clay and was told by many that I was talented. Several years later I studied sculpting at evening classes at the Brooklyn museum. I then moved on from clay into stone sculpting. I took a beginner's class and felt like a bird in flight. I loved the feel of the hammer and chisel carving through the hard stone and the ability to take an amorphous piece of rock and create a beautiful work of art. I have studied under some of the best local sculptors and have made over a dozen sculptures. My pieces have been exhibited in several group shows around the metro area. Even if I never become famous from sculpting, it was a great outlet for me creatively and psychologically.

After practicing medicine for several years I developed a small nest egg which I decided to use to buy art. I contacted Sotheby's, to obtain a catalog for an upcoming auction, and found 10 paintings that I liked. Each one had a high and low estimate. I thought it would be a good idea to put in a bid for 10% above the low estimate on every painting I liked. If my bid was accepted I felt I would be getting art at a bargain. I did not even see the paintings in person but I was ready to take the risk. Again, "a life without risk is not worth living". Thank you Helen Keller! Sotheby's called me several days before the auction to make sure I wanted to enter so many bids since they added up to $250,000. I asked myself, Harvey, what if you have to buy all the pieces? I decided to go ahead take the chance. Luckily, my bids were successful on just four pieces, a Chagall, a Picasso, a Leger, and a Valtat. The paintings were far better in person than in the catalog. I thoroughly enjoyed the proximity and communication with great art. It was the start of something big, and a new passion--art collecting.

I eventually sold the Valtat, but still own the others, which have skyrocketed in value. Not only are they beautiful to look at but they are a great investment. Since then I have added more than fifty paintings and sculptures to my collection with each piece carefully picked for aesthetics and value. Many of them are in art books and several have been borrowed by museums.

With regard to starting my art business, I first had cards made up with the name of my company, "Fine Arts limited". How's that for a non-descript name? I aligned myself with several art galleries in the city and sent out 500 letters to doctors on the staff of hospitals I belonged to. In the letter I introduced myself, although half of them already knew me, and explained how I could help them collect beautiful art and make money at the same time. I waited by the phone for the calls to pour in. To my dismay I received only two replies and did not make a single sale. I was really surprised because the art market was doing extremely well at the time. Doctors are notorious for making bad investments, but here was a golden opportunity. My career as an art dealer ended before it began.

My second career choice was to become a stockbroker. I invested in the market for many years and have done quite well, about 25 % per year. I was making more money in the market than in my practice. Many of my friends and colleagues knew that I was a savvy investor and frequently asked me questions about their own investments. I was getting called on a daily basis for my advice. So why not charge money?

The first step was to obtain a license. I would have to pass the infamous "Series-7" exam. At this stage of my life I thought I was finished taking exams. Not! In order to sit for the exam I had to be sponsored by a brokerage firm, so I called several but they would only sponsor me if I first worked for them for a minimum of a year. Thanks but no thanks! Then I remembered that a patient of mine was an owner of a small firm so I asked him. To my surprise he agreed to sponsor me. I went back to college at C.W. Post to take a review course. Most of the students were younger had majored in business and had MBA's. This was going to be the first test that I had taken in many years and it was given entirely on the computer. I was ready for the challenge and studied my ass off. My ass did not become any smaller but I did score a 90% on the exam. Did this mean I was going to become a successful stockbroker? I worked as a broker for about three days, part-time, and then realized this was not for me. Cold calling and kissing up to prospective clients was not my style. The main problem was that I did not want to be responsible for other people's money especially when the market takes a turn for the worse. Everybody loves you when the market goes up but you are despised when it goes down. It has to be one of the most stressful jobs in the world. Surgery is a cakewalk compared to this. My stockbroker career ended quite rapidly but it was a great learning experience and I did have fun while it lasted.

After striking out twice, I began to appreciate orthopedics more and realized that I had a terrific job in the best location and should not take it for granted. I focused more energy on my practice than ever before. I even walked in to my office with a smile on my face. I accepted and began to appreciate the fact that I was a successful orthopedist. After all, somebody has to do it. Now that I have resolved that problem, my next goal was to find my soulmate and then my life would be complete.

Right after I moved out of my house, I met Susan. I was at a singles party at the Barbazon Hotel in NYC. She was every man's dream— beautiful, sexy, sophisticated, smart, and successful. She was a femme fatale and always the center of attention. I struck up a conversation and asked what kind of work she did. She told me she was a cosmetologist (a fancy name for a make-up artist, usually an uneducated bimbo). I knew she was lying but went along with it and said "how nice " and that she must be very talented. I knew she was testing me but it showed me that she was not only a liar, but also a snob with an attitude. Was this her attempt at humor? If she could lie then so could I, so I told her I was an art dealer. Sometimes it gets boring to tell people that I am an orthopedic surgeon over and over again. But it was not a complete lie since I do buy and sell paintings, which technically makes me a dealer. Eventually she told me her real job, a personal trainer, and an owner of a small exercise studio. I should have known since she was in excellent shape. She told me her name was Susan, so I started calling her Sue. She quickly corrected me and told me not to call her Sue, since she had an aunt with that name that she did not like. I was not impressed with this explanation. She was the only Susan I had ever met who didn't like being called Sue, but I complied with her wish anyway. What did impress me were her petite, bouncy manner, her sexy raspy voice, and her big blue eyes. I took the bait-- hook, line and sinker, and had an exciting roller coaster ride for 3 1/2 years.

She was a personal trainer for the movers and shakers of NYC. Her Rolodex was a virtual who's who in the city. She trained the likes of Tina Brown, Oprah Winfrey, Jackie O, and others. She introduced me to a new world that was connected and exciting. I attended parties with famous celebrities and felt like a celebrity myself, just by being in their company. It was also fun to brag about whom I met. At one amazing party I met Madonna, Cindy Crawford and David Bowie. But there was one tiny problem--my girlfriend was a walking terror. Aside from being mean, selfish, argumentative, and stubborn, she was perfect. She knew exactly how to push my buttons and I don't mean the good ones. Despite the problems I tried to be optimistic and hoped things would improve and she would change. I even hoped that I would change so we could get along better.

After three years I bought her a beautiful diamond engagement ring that she wore for about two weeks. Then I received the famous phone call. She was riding on the bus when someone pick-pocketed her purse where she just happened to be keeping the ring. The ring was stolen! I did not believe the story for a minute but I could not prove anything so I accepted it. I knew the relationship was doomed from then on. The sad part is that she knew it before I did and outsmarted me. She scammed the scammer. The ring is probably still sitting in her safety deposit vault.

Just about the time that I broke up with Susan and was feeling very depressed, I am in my office one day, opening the mail. There is a letter from the State Health Department. It was a long letter so first I skimmed through it. I could not believe what I was reading. Before I jumped to any conclusions I read it more carefully a second time. I thought, what the hell is going on here? The state accused me of gross negligence and incompetence on six cases and was going to suspend my license. I was in shock. I know I had a lot of malpractice cases but there were good explanations for each. Where did they get my name? Then I remembered that 5 years ago they asked to review over 20 of my charts. I never heard anything from them since. If I was so incompetent then why did they let me continue to practice for all these years? This was a complete disaster. I was in my late forties at the peak of my career and they wanted to take away my license? I was already very depressed about the breakup with my girlfriend and now I had to deal with the possible end of my career. I literally started to shake. My world was crumbling. I was getting pummeled. I completely lost my self-confidence. My spirit was broken, I could not sleep, and did not want to wake up or get out of bed in the morning. I lost 15 pounds because I couldn't eat. I wished I had never become a doctor.

I contacted several lawyers to see if they could help and eventually hired two whom seemed friendly, receptive to my plight, and competent. Although it would be more costly, I felt that a second lawyer could not hurt and indeed might help. I insisted that I treated these patients properly and that the State had no grounds to take this action. I knew that my lawyers were not convinced until two orthopedic experts reviewed the charts and agreed with me that I had done nothing wrong. Now that I had my lawyers convinced, it was their job to convince the State lawyers. The problem was that once allegations are made it is extremely difficult to get them reversed. After a year of meetings and discussions we did finally convince them that they made a mistake. I maintained my license but was put on probation. This was a huge victory, but the whole ordeal gave me "agita", gray hairs and forced me to double up on Prozac.

During this extremely depressing time I continued my search for a soul mate by placing an ad in New York Magazine. It went something like this "handsome, fit, romantic, sports doctor seeks sexy, sophisticated, sassy lady for romance and long term relationship". I received about 200 replies almost all of them totally unsuitable. The letters came in from all over the country but I was only interested in somebody from the N.Y. area. I was very picky. Finally, I opened one of the last letters and looked at the picture. She was a cross between Candice Bergen and a pussycat, beautiful and cute at the same time. I read the letter, which stated that she was a lawyer, loved cats and art, and would try anything once but if necessary would give it a second chance. She sounded terrific. The next step was to speak with her on the phone. Her name was Ava and although she had a nasal tone to her voice she had such a nice laugh that it did not bother me. We decided to meet the next day in the City. I arrived at the bar early so I could have a few drinks to loosen me up. The drinks worked in two ways. It made me more relaxed and witty and it made the other person look and sound better as well. She walked in and the room lit up. She was even better looking than her picture and had a terrific aura. Her smile was infectious and she loved to laugh. It is especially important for a woman to laugh at a man's jokes even if they are not funny. We chatted for hours and I asked her out for the weekend and to accompany me to New Orleans the following month. She agreed to both. I guess she liked me as much as I liked her. She later admitted that as soon as she saw me she knew she would marry me. We did eventually get engaged and planned to be married, but a funny thing happened along the way.

I planned to have the ceremony at the Belvedere Castle in Central Park (a storybook setting at an old Gothic castle) and the reception at the Plaza Hotel. I thought, it doesn't get any better than this. Several weeks before the wedding we still needed a clergy to officiate and sign the marriage license. I looked through the phone book and found Laura, a clergy and counselor who knew how to perform a Jewish wedding. Of course she wanted to meet with us before the event. We met at her home and within minutes of sitting down Ava and myself started having an argument ranging from the pre-nuptial disagreement to everything else we could conjure up. Laura tried to help us resolve the issues but to no avail. Finally she said that she would not feel comfortable signing the marriage license and suggested that we go for counseling before we got married. Since the invitations had already been sent she suggested that we go ahead with the party but change the occasion from a "marriage" to a "commitment towards marriage" ceremony. Rightfully so, she felt we should worked out our differences before signing the contract.

We had the party and it was terrific despite the fact that everybody was confused and nobody knew what they were celebrating. We went on a "honeymoon" to Spain and Las Vegas. Shortly after we returned we went out on a Saturday night with a group of my friends to a disco and restaurant. Everybody was having a good time drinking dancing and eating. While I was dancing with another woman (it was common in our group to switch dancing partners) I playfully pinched her backside. Ava saw me, and all hell broke loose. She became irate and wanted to leave the party immediately. Although I apologized for my behavior and explained that I was just being playful but she did not care. We went home and slept it off. The next morning the argument started all over again. I told her I did not want to fight and that I was going out to jog and would be back in thirty minutes. When I returned I was astonished to see that Ava had packed all her belongings and was going to leave. I tried to convince her not to go but she had already made up her mind. I could not believe this was happening only one month after our "honeymoon". After she left I called her many times but she refused to answer the phone or return my calls. Several weeks later she agreed to meet at Laura's office but was still very angry and not willing to forgive or forget. The relationship was over. I tried calling her several more times. It was over. Once again I felt like a failure, rejected and alone. Combined with everything else, the winter of 2000 was one of the lowest points of my life.

When I am making money my other problems seem less important and for the previous five years the stock market was on a bull- run. In 1999 the NASDAQ market consisting of technology stocks had its best year ever and the value of my portfolio tripled. I watched CNBC business news religiously and it seemed like I was making money every day. I was on my way to becoming a billionaire. Unfortunately, the bubble burst in 2000 and wiped out all my gains from the previous year. This was one of the worst bear markets in history. Everyday my portfolio was losing money. Each time it looked like there was going to be a turnaround and I put money back in, the market would go south. A famous guru said to buy when there was blood in the streets. Not only was there blood, there were body parts, but the bears kept coming. My dream of becoming a billionaire had to be put on hold.

Then comes the final blow. Just when I thought things couldn't get worse, I received a puzzling letter from a journalist for the Daily News. He said he was doing an article about doctors who had a large number of malpractice suits and wanted to question me about my cases. I wrote back and said that the vast majority of my cases were frivolous and explained the reasons why. I told him that I had one of the biggest orthopedic practices on Long Island and handled many difficult cases that other doctors referred to me. Moreover, I was located in the most litigious area in the country and was involved in the most frequently sued specialty. Since I had nothing to hide, I invited him to my office for a personal interview. When he arrived I showed him around and answered all his questions. I also showed him a number of articles I had written for the medical journals and a book that contains many thank you letters from grateful patients. I was hoping he would realize that the number of malpractice suits a doctor gets has nothing to do with his ability or competence. Some of the top orthopods in the city who are well known for performing the most complicated surgery are the ones who are sued the most.

Several months went by and I optimistically thought that maybe he was not going to publish the article. I was sadly mistaken. On a bitterly cold Sunday morning, I woke up and turned on the TV. I saw my picture on the cover of the Daily News being shown on Channel One. The newspaper had written a two-page scathing article with pictures about me. All the explanations I had given the reporter were left out and all the negative allegations were printed. It was extremely biased and written with the sole intent of ruining my reputation. The one saving grace was that in the last paragraph, another orthopedist in the area was quoted as saying, "Doctor Manes treats his patients above the standard of care of the community and is a very competent surgeon". That was the bone he thought he could throw in. to balance the article.

I received calls from friends and relatives from all over the country. It seemed as if everybody I had ever known had read the article and called to reassure me that they did not believe a word, but the damage was done. Even my colleagues called me in sympathy. I lost all my prestige and standing in the community. It seemed the only way I could live this down was to be like Bill Clinton during Monica-gate, and make believe that I was completely unaffected by the article.

As expected, there were immediate repercussions. The next day I was called by the medical center in Queens where I was supposed to see patients and told not to bother coming in. I really could not blame them for firing me. I was front-page news. I walked into my office sheepishly, extremely embarrassed, and feeling like I had let everybody down. My faithful employees having worked for me for many years and believed I was one of the best doctors around now had to answer to their friends and relatives about the article. Maybe I was not as good a doctor as they had believed. Several of my patients immediately cancelled their appointments and their surgery. On the whole my patients did come in and voiced their disapproval of the article and told me I was a terrific doctor. The accolades brought tears to my eyes. I was always confident in my ability and knew that deep down inside I am a good doctor and tried my best to help my patients. The next setback was the hospital administrator who called and told me to give up my ER call for awhile. I walked into the general staff meeting the following week and felt that everyone was talking about me behind my back.

In order to survive, I had to put the article behind me and move on. To help regain perspective, I read several newly published philosophy books that appeared to be written just for me at this moment in my life. "The Consolations of Philosophy" and "Plato Not Prozac" are self help books that apply eternal wisdom to life's difficult problems. Basically, when you learn how other people, especially well known philosophers handled their most difficult conflicts, it helps you resolve your own. I surprised myself that I resorted to philosophy to guide me through this arduous time. I am sure Plato would be duly impressed.

During the next few months while I was trying to get back on track, further setbacks occurred. Several insurance companies dropped me from their panel of doctors. Fortunately, I was able to appeal and convince them that I was indeed a good doctor and their patients were in safe hands. They reversed their positions and put me back on board. The worst repercussion came four months later when I was called by the administrator of the hospital and told that I was suspended from the staff. When I asked why I was told that I improperly treated three patients. After reviewing the charts and finding nothing wrong, (they all healed well), I realized this was not about these patients but about the news article. They just wanted me out. I obtained second and third opinions from other orthopods who all agreed that my care was exemplary. The State also reviewed the charts and found no wrongdoing. I am still waiting for the hospital to reverse their suspension.

I felt like Socrates who was tried for heresy because people in power did not like him and his constant questioning. In case you have forgotten he was the dialectic philosopher who was famous for asking people perplexing questions. In his last statement he told the court that they might as well find him guilty because he planned to continue his inquiries and not change. As you know, eventually he was forced to drink hemlock and died. After his death, the people of Athens realized their grave mistake and he was redeemed and thought to have been a great man. A great dead man.

CHAPTER 7: BORN AGAIN

In summary, the year 2000 was one of the worst in my life. What's ironic is that the year before was one of the best since my practice was strong, the stock market was friendly, and I was engaged. In contrast, in 2000 my practice was contracting, the market crashed and what was supposed to be a wedding ceremony turned out to be a breaking up party. Where is the Prozac when you need it? Having experienced so many ups and downs recently, I think I am starting to become immune.

Right after Ava left my life, in walked a beautiful, brilliant, accomplished, sophisticated gentle and sweet woman who I met through another personal ad. Some would say I didn't learn my lesson. The ad was placed in Dan's Paper, the well-known Hampton's tabloid. I thought that anyone who advertises in this paper must be very cool, and she is. I am trying to show her how to be extremely cool though, just like me. For example, recently I bought her several rings, one silver with onyx, another with hematite beads and the third with rhinestones. She wears them on her index finger and thumb. Is that cool or what! Oh yes! Her name is Chynna but I call her "baby-cakes". She is a warm and affectionate person and has helped me through these trying times. I forgot to mention, she is also an expert on investing, which comes in very handy at the moment.

Am I too old to start another career at this stage in my life? I woke up New Years Day and a revelation came to me. Why not become a lawyer? I could follow in the footsteps of great notables such as Abraham Lincoln and Oliver Wendall Holmes, my ex-wife, daughter, and son-in-law. I am constantly involved in multiple litigation at any one time so it would also allow me to save an enormous sum of money in legal fees. I would continue my orthopedic practice while attending law school part-time. I have been told by many that I would make a great lawyer, and besides not enough people hate me yet! I would not have to practice to support myself so I could pick and choose the cases that I found the most interesting. My most obvious interests include art law, trusts and estates, malpractice and would love to handle class action suits against large corporations like Erin Brockovitch.

The mountain is there and I feel compelled to climb it. Step number one was to take the LSAT. Despite the fact that I took a Princeton review course, I scored the same afterwards as I did on a practice exam before the course and was $1000 poorer. However, my score was high enough to obtain admission to the two schools that I applied to and was even offered a scholarship. I start Hofstra or Touro Law School in the fall. After one semester, I will re-evaluate my decision and if I decide to continue, then move over Johnny Cochran!

So far this year my life has taken a turn for the better, probably because it couldn't have gotten any worse. My practice is slow and steady like the tortoise. I am not in any race but would like to continue for another 10 years. I have a lovely lady in my life that I adore and I think she feels the same about me. Last but not least, I have an opportunity to pursue another challenging career.

My first fifty years has been jam-packed with an amazing variety of events. I would love to say that I have no regrets, but I would have been lying. "You pays your money and youse take your chance". I believe I was blessed with talents that I have tried to develop and use to make the world a better place to live. I had an exciting childhood, and I have been pretty lucky as an adult. I have great parents, married a terrific woman, and have four fantastic kids. I had two interesting relationships and a new one that I am sure will continue to develop. I have enough money (is it ever enough?), and a lot to look forward to including the birth of my first grandchild who is due any minute now.

And then I rode off on my white horse with a beautiful princess to the castle of dreams come true and lived happily ever after.

As a parting thought I leave you with this rhyme

Until my days are over,

Never fill my cup.

There is always something to be learned,

Until I finally grow up.

The End !

P.S. Look for the sequel in 50 years.